Porcupines *to*
POLAR BEARS

Adventures of a
Wildlife Veterinarian

Porcupines *to*
POLAR BEARS

Adventures of a
Wildlife Veterinarian

Jerry Haigh

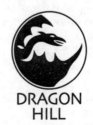

DRAGON
HILL

The Publisher: Dragon Hill Publishing Ltd.
Website: www.dragonhillpublishing.com

Library and Archives Canada Cataloguing in Publication

Haigh, J. C. (Jerry C.), author
Porcupines to polar bears : Adventures of a wildlife veterinarian
/ Jerry Haigh.

Includes bibliographical references.
ISBN 978-1-896124-61-2 (paperback)
ISBN 978-1-896124-62-9 (e-pub)

1. Haigh, J. C. (Jerry C.)—Anecdotes. 2. Wildlife veterinarians—Canada—Anecdotes. I. Title.

SF613.H33A3 2016   636.089092   C2016-900010-9

Project Director: Marina Michaelides
Production & Layout: Tamara Eder
Cover Design: Tamara Eder and Greg Brown
Front Cover Image: Thinkstock images 78740402 and 78740422 © Fuse
Back Cover Image: Tamara Eder
Photo Credits: Every effort has been made to accurately credit the sources of photographs and illustrations. Any errors or omissions should be reported directly to the publisher for correction in future editions.
Most photos courtesy of Jerry Haigh with the following exceptions: Jean Clottes (p. 285); Johane Janelle (p. 267); Manitoba Museum (p. 290); Wes Olson (p. 271, 293); Saskatoon Public Library—Local History (LH-2823) (p. 255); Rob Stewart (pp. 128, 129); Thinkstock (p. 135); Estate of Clarence Tillenius (p. 291, 292).

Produced with the assistance of the Government of
Alberta, Alberta Media Fund.

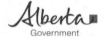

PC:32

Dedication

For Jo, my rock and anchor.

Contents

Introduction 10

CHAPTER 1: New Beginnings 14

CHAPTER 2: Prairie Innocents 22

FIRE ENGINE NUMBER ONE: No Fire, Just Smoke 32

CHAPTER 3: For the Birds! 33

CHAPTER 4: Injections and Pedicures 42

CHAPTER 5: A Near Miss 50

CHAPTER 6: Blowgun Development 52

CHAPTER 7: Captive Bison and Farming. 63

FIRE ENGINE NUMBER TWO: A Small Fire Easily Doused 73

CHAPTER 8: Helicopters at −20° 74

CHAPTER 9: Some Bear Facts 83

CHAPTER 10: A Canoe Trip with a Bonus 94

CHAPTER 11: Hippo Dentistry 102

FIRE ENGINE NUMBER THREE: The Loneliness of the Long
    Distance Owl 112

CHAPTER 12: The Graveyard of the Atlantic. 114

CHAPTER 13: Hooded Seals 125

FIRE ENGINE NUMBER FOUR: A Battering Encounter. 135

CHAPTER 14: A Bear Cub and a Dog 137

CHAPTER 15: Bison Farming. 150

CHAPTER 16: From Farm to Ranch. 159

CHAPTER 17: Tarzan and Family 169

FIRE ENGINE NUMBER FIVE: An Escape with a Bad Ending .. 177

CHAPTER 18: Pond Inlet Part 1: Arrival......................... 178

CHAPTER 19: Pond Inlet Part 2: More Work 187

FIRE ENGINE NUMBER SIX: An Upset Elk.................... 197

CHAPTER 20: A Scary Night 199

FIRE ENGINE NUMBER SEVEN: An Outbreak and
a Remedy.. 209

CHAPTER 21: Return to the Arctic 211

CHAPTER 22: Déjà Vu on an Unusual Lion Case 218

CHAPTER 23: Polar Bear Capital of the World 225

CHAPTER 24: Rubber Bullet: A Traumatic Event 242

FIRE ENGINE NUMBER EIGHT: Vandals at the Zoo 251

CHAPTER 25: Bison Studies in Winter 252

FIRE ENGINE NUMBER NINE: Preventing a Rabies
Outbreak.. 265

CHAPTER 26: Summer Bison 267

FIRE ENGINE NUMBER TEN: A Puzzle Helped by
Laboratory Work 278

CHAPTER 27: Bison in Art 282

CHAPTER 28: A Zoo Society: Yesterday and Today............. 297

Notes on Sources.. 301

Stories, great flapping ribbons of shaped space-time,
have been blowing and uncoiling around the universe since
the beginning of time.
—Terry Pratchett, *Witches Abroad*

Life is what you make it.
—Harry Gordon Selfridge

They should tell you when you're born, have a suitcase heart,
be ready to travel.
—Gabriele Zevin

Acknowledgements

First, more than thanks to my wife, Jo, who read and suggested changes to the manuscript. She encouraged me to start, straightened me out about facts and corrected my many spelling mistakes. She also kept me going when I needed help.

Of course a multitude of thanks to the publisher, Marina Michaelides and to Faye Boer, who approached and encouraged me to write these stories and who introduced me to Dragon Hill Publishing. Other team members were also heavily involved. Wendy Pirk did the proofreading. Tamara Eder was the layout and production artist and Photoshop wizard, (especially to change colour photos to black and white). Finally, Greg Brown, did the cover design and layout.

Then thanks to the many people who helped me with editing, recall, suggestions, and gave permission to use their images in photos. They are Lesley Avant, Susan Blum, Claire Bullaro, Nigel Caulkett, Jean Clottes, Shirley Collinridge, Meaghan Craven, Andy Derocher, Cormack Gates, Stu Hampton, Shannon Harnett, Johane Janelle, Petr Komers, John Lee, Sue Lewis, Murray Lindsay, John MacDonald, Judy McCrosky, Peter and Kay Mehren, Jeanette Montgomery, Jerry Ninuit, Wes Olson, Lily Ootoova, Perry Robinson, Terry Rock, Wayne Runge, Paul Sayer, Sharon Schmidt, Bob Stewart, Rob Stewart, Ray Schweinsburg, Larry Strome, Gerhard Stuewe, Doug Whiteside, Murray Woodbury and Bob Wooley. Also to the late Malcolm Ramsay.

Jean Clottes, Johane Janelle, Wes Olson, Paul Sayer and Rob Stewart had no hesitation in letting me use their own photos and illustrations. Thanks to them as well.

Introduction

L uck. A series of lucky moments. That is what has characterized a 50-year career as a veterinarian.

The luck started in Kenya, where I was born (I had nothing to do with the initiation of this event). My parents were in East Africa during World War II because in 1939 my father, a subaltern in the Highland Light Infantry, was seconded out from Fort George in wet and windy northeastern Scotland. In Kenya he joined the King's African Rifles.

My mother, his fiancé, joined him a few months later. Her five-day journey aboard a Sunderland Flying boat left Southampton and stopped at Marseilles, Alexandria, Khartoum, Juba, Entebbe and at last Kisumu on the shores of Lake Victoria in Kenya. Dad told me she was the last civilian woman allowed to travel to Africa after the declaration of war. They were married at the Cathedral of the

Highlands in Nairobi on December 21, 1939, and 18 months later I arrived.

The next lucky part was indolence on my part—usually not thought to be luck, but it was. The examiners at the Glasgow Veterinary School required me to repeat my second year of studies. Had I graduated as originally planned in 1964, the internship position at the newly minted Kabete Veterinary College just outside Nairobi would not have been available. I applied and was accepted.

Perhaps the most amazing stroke of luck was the fact that I could play a respectable game of tennis, which needs some clarification.

Three days after the graduation ceremony in Glasgow, I boarded a British Overseas Airways Corporation Comet 4 for the long trip to Nairobi. My former classmate and 1964 graduate, Jimmy Duncan met me at the airport. We hadn't been driving for five minutes when he informed me that he had entered me into a tennis tournament that same evening. After the tennis, and over a beer in the clubhouse, I met some of the other players, including blond, tough-looking Tony Parkinson.

So it turned out that six days after graduation, and wet behind the ears, I was on duty for the Large Animal Clinic field service when Tony called for someone to come to his compound to deal with a lame giraffe. Tony was a zoological collector in partnership with his godfather, John Seago. It was my first wildlife case.

Because we'd had a shortage of giraffes in Glasgow in 1965, I applied first principles: approach the case as if the animal was just an overgrown cow, another ruminant. It was quickly obvious that the giraffe was suffering from a condition called foul of the foot or foot rot. Either name is graphic enough to need no detailed description. Vets and cattle farmers know it well. The main challenge for me was injecting the penicillin into his backside far above my head. He recovered.

After that, more "normal" cases involving cattle, horses and later dogs and cats were daily fare. Two tame cheetahs showed up at the small animal clinic, causing some excitement. One had a case of worms, easily treated. The other involved the fracture of both hind legs. An orthopedic surgeon from Nairobi Hospital helped with this complicated case.

Eighteen months later, after a short spell in England but having caught the Africa bug, I was back in Kenya working as District Veterinary Officer based in the small market town of Meru. The main challenge was dealing with thousands of cattle and the inevitable load of bureaucracy. Eight dogs and one horse were the other patients in four years.

A year into my posting came a pivotal moment, a tipping point if you will. Maybe it was luck again, just being in the right place at the right time. Peter Jenkins, the warden at Meru Game Park, asked me to examine a sick rhino, and over the course of the next three years I tended to a few more similar cases in the park. They were not truly wild animals. They had been imported from southern Africa, where they had been raised in captivity as part of a conservation program. Word obviously got out that here was a vet willing to treat rhinos and other wild animals.

That first-day tennis tournament came to roost. Tony Parkinson called to ask if I would join the team in a translocation effort where rhinos were to be moved from a new settlement area to various national parks, including Meru.

Four years after starting the government job and now married to Jo (the love of my life) and with a small daughter, I opened a clinic 80 kilometres (50 miles) 'round the base of Mount Kenya in the town of Nanyuki. While

I worked in the clinic, Jo set up her medical practice at the Nanyuki Cottage Hospital. On top of domestic animal work, I had the enormous good fortune (more luck) to have Don Hunt as a wildlife client. His collection at the Mount Kenya Game Ranch required frequent attention, often in the form of health certificates for export. In addition, he made several trips to capture rhinos, elephants and giraffes.

By this time I had some idea of what I was doing. So nine years after that first rhino patient in Meru and after helping relocate more than 100 rhinos to what was then considered safety, I was offered the position at Saskatoon's Western College of Veterinary Medicine as a zoo and wildlife specialist. No exams and no formal academic postgraduate qualifications were required. All I needed was a few glowing letters of reference and a serendipitous visit by my former dean at Glasgow, Sir William Weipers, to Saskatoon while candidate deliberations were in progress. These days no one could hope to land a job like that without serious post-graduate study and some sort of specialist training.

For the next 33 years I was immersed in the routine and not-so-routine challenges of the politics of a university and a small zoo. In the latter I dealt with dental problems for a lion and a hippo as well as two mysteries in porcupines. Even more exciting was the chance to criss-cross my new country and work on free-ranging wild animals such as moose, seals, bison and polar bears. What follows is a collection of stories about the animals and people I encountered during those years.

CHAPTER 1

New Beginnings

Where to start? That's the big question I asked myself as I sat in the buffeteria on the second floor of the Western College of Veterinary Medicine. Nibbling on a peanut butter cookie, cup of tea in hand, I tried to imagine what challenges lay ahead. At this time of day a month earlier I had been in the Marina café across the road from my office in Kenya on Nanyuki's main street. After a brief stop in Europe to visit family, I arrived in Saskatoon to start my new job as a zoo and wildlife veterinarian.

And I had more than one question than just where to start. What to do first in the zoo? And then subsequently? These were the problems.

One positive note, a large Chevrolet Impala had been set aside for my exclusive use. It was almost double in size of any saloon I had driven before, big enough to seem as if it had an engine at both ends but not as big as my imagined Yellow Submarine. It was sort of mustard yellow colour and had seen better days. But it ran well and that was what mattered.

Learning to drive on the wrong side of the road was another challenge.

The move from the slopes of Mount Kenya to the prairies of Saskatchewan was a huge change. My new home had no hills let alone mountains.

Sometimes, in my mind's eye I could still see the African mountain's three jagged peaks, each named for a Maasai chief. They often looked as if they were enveloped by a bride's veil of wispy clouds. During the rainy season the peaks could only be imagined behind huge, dark banks of cloud. Most dramatic of all, when skies were clear, the glaciers and snowy peaks were pristine and stunning. In many countries the weather is the opening gambit to any conversation. In Nanyuki, it was the mountain.

Farther up the slopes of the mountain was the Mount Kenya Safari Club, an up-market hotel with an impressive collection of birds that I had to treat from time to time.

Adjacent to the club was the Mount Kenya Game Ranch. The owners were film star William Holden, safari guide and hunter Julian McKeand and TV star Don Hunt and his wife Iris, who lived on the ranch.

The collection of larger creatures included zebras, a couple of giraffes and a considerable collection of antelopes, all the way from tiny dikdik to the largest of all in Africa, the pale brown, spiral horned eland.

Perhaps the most beautiful of these were a few mountain bongo. They too had spiral horns, but their most striking feature was the rich chocolate hide with its series of creamy-yellow stripes on each side.

They were held in a fenced compound along with a group of injured crowned cranes. I often had to capture

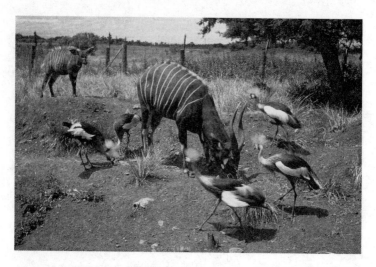

A bongo bull feeds from a trough while crowned cranes wait their turn.

several of the antelopes for transfer to the quarantine hold-ings in the port of Mombasa. There I had to test them again to ensure that they had no disease they might carry with them to other countries, usually the U.S.

Among the oddest-looking of the creatures on the ranch was the wildebeest, which needed frequent intervention. Of course the wildebeest is best known for the yearly mass migration that takes place between Tanzania's Serengeti National Park and the open plains of the Maasai Mara across the border into Kenya. I cannot think of a single African documentary that fails to show graphic footage of the masses of wildebeest in their desperate driven urge to cross the Mara River and the hungry crocodiles in the water anticipating a wildebeest meal. The other story of wildebeest that is less gruesome and is part of folklore is the notion that they were the last creatures created by Ngai, the God of several tribes in East Africa. Legend has it that they are made up of spare parts left over from other

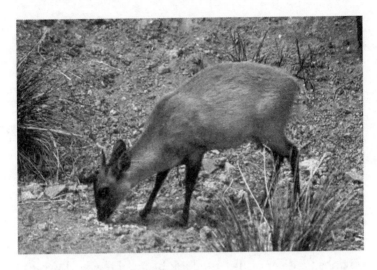

A duiker at the Mt. Kenya Game Ranch

efforts. They have the face of a turtle, the ears of a fox, the beard and mane of a lion, the horns of a buffalo, the body of a cow, the legs of an antelope and the tail of a horse.

Other wild creatures at the ranch included elephants, rhinos, cheetahs, leopards and even lemurs that came from Madagascar. Lemurs have two distinguishing characteristics. They are less intelligent than pigeons in some tests and they have a vicious bite, as Iris discovered to her cost.

A more limited area of the ranch housed a collection of birds such as wing-damaged owls and an augur buzzard that were brought in by concerned members of the public.

The saddest resident at the ranch was an adult male chimpanzee named Jonjon. He had arrived as a tiny infant. Iris fell for him at once and took over the responsibility of raising him. In due course he had grown into a powerful adult but was impossible to handle or trust. He became downright dangerous and demonstrated his infatuation for Iris by getting a hard-on whenever he saw her.

Early claims from experiments carried out in the 1920s were that chimps are five times as strong as humans. Although it might take five men to subdue one because of its agility, the truth is that in terms of real strength, the figure is actually double.

Five or two, the figure hardly matters. When I first met Jonjon, he had a padlocked chain around his neck. The other end of the 15-metre-long (50-foot) chain was padlocked around the base of a large umbrella acacia. This gave him enough freedom to clamber up into the fork of the tree or move in a circle around its base.

Most of the time he looked thoroughly unhappy as he sat scowling in the fork. The first time I visited, it was obvious he did not like the look of me. He was down on the ground in a flash and charged. It was a scary moment. My first thought was "will the chain hold." Luckily it did. When visitors came to the ranch and got too close, he would not only charge but hurl things at them. Sticks were not too dangerous, but his dung was a nastier weapon. And he was accurate, no doubt as a result of long practice.

Members of the staff were usually careful around him. His food was thrown to him from well outside his perimeter. But one day Julius, a slim keeper with a distinctive scar on his arm, was tidying up the sticks and other less savoury material lying around. He got too close when he tried to pick up some of the debris. The chimp came at him in full charge mode, teeth bared, screaming, with a face like thunder.

Like any of us who have no desire to be torn limb from limb, Julius used one of the sticks he had picked up and threw it. By a horrific piece of bad luck, the stick flew right into the ape's left eye. The accident no doubt saved Julius from a mauling, or worse. The chimp had no such luck.

John, a tall, handsome Kikuyu who was the manager of the collection, called me right away. John's tone of voice was enough to indicate that his was a genuine emergency. Into the workhorse Peugeot 404 wagon, sandwich in hand, and I was off up the hill.

From 18 metres (60 feet) I could see no details. Even a look through binoculars did not give me much more information. What next?

Don was in Nairobi so we couldn't do any more until I spoke to him. He called the next morning and at once asked me to do what I could for Iris' favourite animal.

I needed to take closer look, but how? I had my new dart gun with me because I never knew on visits to the ranch what might come next. The gun, while fairly accurate was not a precision instrument. At a range of 10 metres (33 feet) I could not be sure of hitting the chimp's backside. A hit in any other area carries a severe risk of either breaking a bone or burying itself in some sensitive area like the belly or over the lower back into a kidney. Unfortunately, Jonjon would not turn around and present the required target. He was more interested in the possibility of having a go at me. Chimps are known to rip the testes from their victims—not a fate at the top of my bucket list. In fact, it is not on the list at all.

John suggested that I might be able to put the drug I needed into an orange and offer that to Jonjon. "He loves oranges." So that is what we did.

The chimp took no time at all to swallow the Trojan horse. In 10 minutes he began to show signs of being drowsy. We waited a further 10 minutes before he fell onto his side. Even then nobody was going to get inside his perimeter until we could be sure it was safe.

The chimp's eye was badly damaged; the stick had destroyed the eyeball. I could see no sign of infection, so

I elected to give him an injection of antibiotic into the socket and hope that things would be okay. Two days later it was obvious they were not. The remnants of the damaged eye had to come out.

The relatively simple surgery was not the main challenge. Anesthesia was a different kettle of fish. This time, Jonjon would have nothing to do with the proffered orange. The drug I used the first time was a powerful hallucinogenic. It is a recreational drug with more than 20 street names.

Recreational is a gross misnomer as there are plenty of horror stories of people who have misused the drug. I read about one young man who tore his own eyes out under the influence. In another report, a man threw himself down an elevator shaft because he thought he could fly. One would certainly not want to take the drug unintentionally or even splash a drop or two into one's eyes or mouth.

There is no way of knowing what sorts of hallucinations Jonjon suffered while under the influence. He must have smelled the stuff in the second orange and decided it was not for him. No elevator shafts, thank you very much!

John suggested a dose of whisky. What a sad reflection of Jonjon's life that he had developed a liking for alcohol! So with no other alternative, Julius offered a doctored bottle, which he shoved toward the chimp with a long stick. Jonjon downed the concoction in three gulps.

The surgery was over in 20 minutes. The most delicate part of the operation was the placement of five buried sutures. The last thing any of us needed was for Jonjon to pick at tag ends and pull them out. An injection of antibiotic completed the medical part of the event. Jonjon's recovery was a different matter, however. It took him six hours to come round. When he had fully recovered, he seemed less upset about his eye. At least it appeared I had done *some* good.

During my time in Kenya, I dealt with more than 100 rhinos, numerous elephants and a lame giraffe. As for carnivores, while I was an intern at the vet college, I assisted in the repair of two broken legs on a tame cheetah. Another cheetah patient was Joy Adamson's Pippa that had weak bones due to the all-meat diet she was fed. Such a diet lacks calcium, which leads to bone abnormalities including fractures. Joy is best known for both her art and her conservation work. *Born Free* (both a book and a movie) describes her experiences raising a lion cub named Elsa. She later published *Pippa's Challenge*, the story of her cheetah. She didn't mention the suggestion of a diet change. She probably took no notice.

Another Kenya client, Mr. Court Parfet, the American chewing gum millionaire, owned the country's first private game ranch. I visited the ranch to deal with a sick lion and also helped with the capture and treatment of rhinos.

Three years later, when Don Hunt heard about our upcoming departure for Canada, he asked me to euthanize Jonjon before I left. The chimp had become too dangerous, and his nasty habit of dung throwing had escalated. Don also said that the keepers, particularly John, were attached to the old rascal, so he asked me to pretend that the chimp was being transferred to a place where he could be better handled. I am fairly certain that nobody believed a word of that piece of fiction, but the deed was done.

The experiences gained with this wide variety of animals stood me in good stead in my new post with the University of Saskatchewan, even if the species were new to me.

CHAPTER 2

Prairie Innocents

S uddenly, I was on the Canadian prairies. What a change!

The morning drive to Saskatoon's newish zoo under the influence of jet lag was an interesting experience. At the zoo, my first case was a failure when a darted deer died within the hour. I hoped such a bad start would not be a sign of future misfortunes. As it turned out, the anesthetic merely hastened the animal's end and possibly saved it some suffering as the post mortem showed that it was riddled with cancer.

Over and above all the wildlife cases I treated in Africa, my previous experience of what, in the strictest sense, a modern zoo involved was limited to one visit. That took place in Munich, Germany, on my way from Kenya to Canada at my first international conference—the Wildlife Disease Association, which met at the university. Dr. Ole Nielsen, dean of the WCVM offered to cover my costs if

I attended the conference on my way to my new position in Saskatchewan. It was an offer I could not refuse.

Many interesting people from several different countries were at the gathering. Most were helpful and welcoming, but one sticks in my mind more than 40 years later. As we quaffed our beers in their traditional decorated steins at the reception hosted by the city's mayor, he said, "Ah, you're the guy who got that job in Saskatoon. I've always wanted to meet someone going there. I know several who have left, you are the first I've met going to Saskatoon." His bearded face appears in my mind's eye as I write. While I was still wondering what on earth he meant, he grinned and thus gave away his leg-pull.

During the conference, all the delegates spent an after-noon at the city zoo. The contrast between the memory of that visit and what I saw before me in my new situation was stark.

In Germany there were masses of mature trees, curved paths, clever use of landscaping and several moats that gave the impression of space separation for the outdoor exhibits. In Saskatchewan I saw few mature trees, and every one of the outdoor pens that held deer, sheep, bison and other hoofed stock was laid out in a geometric pattern much like a city block.

Whoever designed the layout may have been a fine town planner, but they had no idea of natural animal space. While this may not have mattered except in the aesthetic sense, the town planner took that experience to the nth degree by placing every animal shelter right in the centre of each pen, thus ensuring there was no way of handling any of the animals should they need medical attention or to be rounded up for transfer to another place. The layout nicely matched the paradigm of "the ideal family home" in Saskatoon, with the single family dwelling in the middle of a garden. The right angle corners, straight lines and 2-metre (7-foot) page wire fences resembled natural animal habitats about as much as a motorcycle resembles a cardboard box.

There was one thing I could do little about. The entire area was completely flat as, of course, is much of the province. The only changes in elevation were the 3-metre (10-foot) tall animal shelters and piles of rock in two pens occupied by mountain sheep that at least gave the impression of an attempt at natural habitat.

With so many things beyond the terrain to think about, I realized it would take time and patience to get them all done. It was a bit like climbing a mountain; I could not accomplish all I wanted to in one day—one step at a time, with rest stops.

In this reflective mood I chatted with the zoo foreman, red-haired, red-bearded Brent Pendleton. He was a Saskatoon resident and had taken some courses to learn his trade. We had to set priorities on what were the most pressing needs. The animals had had no routine veterinary services at all. There were vaccinations to think about, dietary matters and no doubt other standard tasks that a vet would need to deal with. As I walked around, I could see that the sheep and other hoofed stock had overgrown feet that would soon need attention. On top of those were the "fire-engine" cases.

In 1964 the city council of the day closed down an old zoo-type operation called the Golden Gate. They purchased some of the animals and equipment and moved them across the city to the Forestry Farm, which had been an important silviculture (tree production and management) site for the province since 1913.

On viewing some old faded slides of the Golden Gate, I could describe it, if feeling charitable, only as a nasty roadside menagerie. Of course, with an extensive background of free-ranging, wild animals in Kenya I was biased, but those photos were depressing. Open-sided shelters for deer looked like the aftermath of bombings. One of the plywood sheets in a deer pen appeared to have been chomped on by a large carnivore, something about the size of a *T. rex*. The nastiest image of all was of a mangy-looking cat crouched inside a wooden crate the size of a large suitcase, looking out through the mesh. The sign above the crate stated: "Do not tease the animals." Huh?!

The dramatic image in the collection of slides was of a man clad in cowboy hat and boots, throwing a lariat, as a fully antlered fallow deer ran in full gallop beneath it. The photographer, in pre-digital, repeat-shutter days was either very skilled or incredibly lucky. The picture, worth at least a couple of thousand words, spoke volumes about the man's remarkable skills with the rope. It also indicated a great deal about his poor management and lack of any feeling for animal welfare.

The new animal park opened in 1972, three years before my arrival, and any veterinary work had been carried out on an *ad hoc* basis by whomever could find the time or had some of the necessary skills. New, much larger pens had been built for the hoofed stock, and the carnivores were accommodated in much more reasonable, although far from perfect, enclosures.

The dingo cage in Saskatoon was almost certainly a carry-over from the Golden Gate. It was a totally inadequate, wood-framed wire cage with a footprint of about 4 by 4 metres (13 by 13 feet) and just less than 2 metres (7 feet) high.

A much-chewed wooden box just big enough for both animals sat on a shelf in one corner. It was an eyesore, not in the least helped by the information sign with stencilled

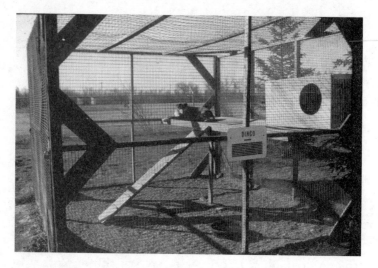

Not the best pen in the zoo

lettering attached to one of the posts. It was illegible, as were the other signs around the grounds.

When I mentioned the unsuitable pen to a senior city hall administrator responsible for the whole transfer exercise, he replied, "Oh, I like that display best of all."

Oh dear! He was my boss on the city side of the appointment. If the occupants really were dingoes, how they got from "Down Under" to the Canadian prairies was a complete mystery.

The pen for the two lions was marginally better. It consisted of an octagonal enclosure about 10 metres (33 feet) across surrounded by a chain-link fence about 4 metres (13 feet) high, with an overhang to the inside. Outside that was a 1-metre (3-foot) restraining fence, presumably but ineffectively designed to keep the public and the big cats apart.

I was at once reminded of the monologue "Albert and the Lion," which I knew best from the wonderful telling

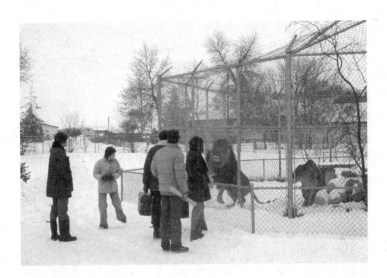

The lions in winter

by Stanley Holloway. In that story, young Albert is pulled into the lion cage and swallowed whole when he annoys Wallace, the lion, by poking his "stick with the orse's ead andle" into its ear.

Visitors, including fairly young children, could easily reach across and endanger themselves or harm the lions using a stick with a horse's head or other similar objects such as a hockey stick (seeing as we were in Canada).

Over to one side, a concrete culvert about 1.5 metres (5 feet) in diameter with metal trap doors at either end provided the only shelter. The enclosure was not heated in any way, although, as I found out when September's Indian summer turned to December's freeze-up, some straw was thrown into the culvert during winter months.

There were also a wide variety of hoofed animals, or hoof stock, mostly native to Canada, although the Japanese sika deer, South American guanacos and dwarf Sicilian donkeys were obviously not. All these species were new to me, but the novelty made for interesting possibilities as my new job began to unfold.

Living out in the dozen or so large pens were four native deer species and three pens of fallow deer. Something of an anomaly in the deer world, fallow deer come in a variety of colours ranging from white to spotted to black. They originated in the Middle East and around the Mediterranean but have been translocated to many corners of the world, including South Africa, in the last two thousand years. The Romans took them to Britain in the first century CE, where the deer thrived, and they have since flourished all over North America.

The native deer included white-tailed deer, mule deer and elk, as well as caribou that looked like the red-nosed reindeer called Rudolph of the Christmas song.

Pens also held three species of wild sheep, and in the largest pen of all were those iconic Canadian animals, the dark brown, shaggy bison. Their huge heads and powerful bodies were a reminder of the Cape buffalo in Africa.

Rodents were represented by three species. The porcupines spent most of the daylight hours with their heads jammed into a dark corner of the box that had been built for them. The group of captive black-tailed prairie dogs were housed in a concrete-walled pen with walls low enough to permit young children to peer over the edge and delight in the cheeky looks as the little creature's heads popped up from their burrows. The pen was lined with excavation-proof netting to prevent the little guys from tunnelling out.

Huge numbers of Richardson's Ground Squirrels, more commonly known as gophers, had invaded the grounds and could be seen almost anywhere. When undisturbed they sat on top of little mounds of excavated earth and looked cheekily at any passing human. They were so used to us that they didn't bother to run away unless someone got too close. If they saw hawks or other birds of prey flying overhead, they let out a short, low-pitched chirps, and the entire colony vanished into their burrows.

The porcupines seemed to subsist on branches thrown into their pen each day. Although the branches were not disturbed during daylight hours, they were always stripped of bark when the keepers arrived in the morning.

Another thing must have occurred at night. In the spring a tiny replica, quills and all, of the parents appeared in the pen, much to everyone's delight and surprise. Naturally, wondered how these well-armed creatures "got it on."

The question stimulated a search. A bizarre and highly improbable explanation comes from the journals of Samuel Hearne. Hearne is best known as the first Caucasian to reach the Arctic Ocean overland, but he was much more than that. One of Hearne's passions was natural history, and he recorded many interesting observations. In the case of the sexual activity of porcupines, he was spectacularly wrong. In one of his many books, Stewart Houston, retired University of Saskatchewan professor and avid historian, he wrote that Hearne "represents an interesting combination of physical endurance and intellectual curiosity." Houston suspects that Hearne may have relied on First Nations hearsay rather than his own observation. Hearne wrote:

> *Their mode of copulation is singular for their quills will not permit them to perform that office in the usual mode, like other quadrupeds. To remedy this inconvenience, they sometimes lie on their sides and meet in that manner; but the usual mode is for the male to lie on his back, and the female to walk over him (beginning at his head), till the parts of generation come into contact.*

Sounds to me like a porcupine version of 69 gone slightly wrong.

Houston further states:

> *Such misconceptions* [he assures me that this was not a pun] *persisted for nearly two centuries after Hearne. The fact is that a few days prior to copulation, the porcupines will meet, belly to belly, as part of their courting procedure.*

As we walked around and chatted, Brent filled me in on the other zoo staff. It was soon obvious that there was a dearth of zookeeper experience. John and Jureen, the two oldest and both near retirement age, had come across from the Golden Gate on the west end of the city. They were entitled to because of union seniority. Both were born in the 1930s, the years known in the prairies as the "Dirty Thirties" partly because of the severe drought that hit the region. The dry soil was picked up and blown away. The half-true saying was that the topsoil from Saskatchewan ended up in Manitoba, the province immediately to the east. This makes sense because the prevailing wind comes from the west.

Those difficult times are seared into the very fabric of Saskatchewan history and have spawned novels, plays and other works of art. The most famous novel is *Who Has Seen The Wind*, written by W.O. Mitchell in 1947, which depicts the life of a boy growing up during those brutal years. When I requested it, the city librarian had no trouble pulling a copy from the shelves. It is a wonderful read that gave me a real taste of how things had been in my new home.

Both John and Jureen had left school to help on the farm after only a few years of schooling—grade two in Jureen's case. He was from a time when many children had to do the same. Neither man had much book learning, but both had lots of animal experience.

Harold Kinsel, a middle-aged man with a solid figure, came from a farming background as well and had dealt with livestock. The youngest staff member was enthusiastic, but also the least experienced. Stuart Hampton, known as Stu, was an extrovert with a wide smile, a ready wit and a good dose of satire.

He recently told me, "I got the job because of my hunting experience. I can tell a mallard from a pintail duck in flight. I know the difference between a mule deer and a white-tailed deer." He was keen to learn, and he read lots of books.

At coffee time we all sat with Brent and discussed the challenges facing us. Many things needed attention, but it would be impossible to make wholesale alterations all at once. Because not a single creature had ever been vaccinated, that was the first priority. We all agreed that the carnivores in the collection should top the list.

These coffee and midday sessions soon had me realizing how different my life would be as I settled in to this new environment.

No Fire, Just Smoke

The porcupines slipped almost out of mind until the foreman decided to move them to a new and more interesting enclosure.

Initially I was not involved, not until a volunteer asked me take a look at the male. It was easy enough to turn him over, wearing gloves, of course. I found a healing wound on the underside of his neck. It looked as if he had been strangled. The wound was a straight line stretching from one ear to the other, vanishing just where the quills grew in.

None of us had any idea what had caused it or where the injury had happened. Our best guess was that he had tried to get out of the enclosure, become trapped part way through the wire mesh and pulled back. The wire probably cut into his flesh before he pulled hard enough to back out.

As for treatment, the healing was well advanced. There was no blood, no pus, no crusting. The only remedy, as much to assuage the concerns of us humans as to do any good for the animal, was to use a purple spray over the wound and let him rejoin his companion in the new enclosure.

CHAPTER 3

For the Birds!

One of the delights of my morning rounds each day was spending time around the several ponds on the zoo grounds.

In that first September and October, a steady flow of migrating wild birds planed in like landing gliders with their wheels down to join our resident waterfowl. They were on their way south for the winter. Mallards, teal and pintails were at once familiar. Redhead ducks and coots looked to be close cousins of the European pochards and coots. Others, such as the smart canvasback with his flat head that reminded me of the caps much favoured by Yorkshire miners in the 1970s, were new to me.

The Canada and white-fronted geese were also new, but a look in the well-worn office copy of *Birds of Canada* made identification an easy task. Other birds in the collection were victims of vehicle encounters and had been earth-bound due to wing damage.

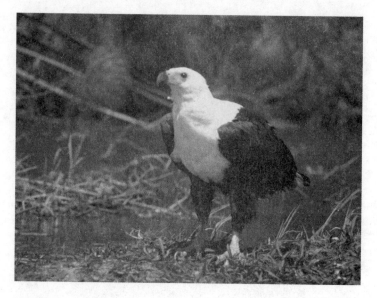

The bib on the African fish eagle makes it easy to distinguish from its American cousin.

Pairs or singles of seven species of raptors occupied several pens. The most majestic was the bald eagle, which I had never seen before. They are remarkably similar to the African fish eagle that I know well. The only easily noted difference is the lack of a chest bib on the North American species. Their haunting cries at once made me think of the sounds of Africa.

The most striking of the five owl species was the great grey owl, with the enormous feathered rings around its eyes. A great horned and two snowy owls were also part of the injured group. Other commonly seen summer residents were red-tailed and Swainson's hawks. All raptors except the eagles and snowy owls were housed in a multi-sided building with outside pens.

Someone with imagination added to the atmosphere in the pen housing the long-eared owl. A yellow Canadian

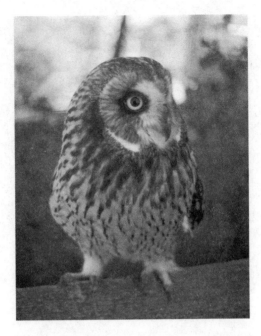

This short-eared owl was one of several raptors that was not able to fly.

Wildlife Service "No Shooting" sign was fixed to a tree stump. It must have been found in an abandoned refuge, but it fitted the theme pretty well.

Wandering the grounds at will were peafowl, the national bird of India, the males strutting their stuff with their amazing multi-eyed tails. Turkeys also strutted their stuff, but could not vie with the peafowl for looks. The Kiswahili term for a turkey is *bata mzinga*, which translates to stupid duck. Right on!

Eventually, Brent and I developed a routine. We knew that plenty of things needed attention. It was just a matter of getting them done one by one as well as dealing with any urgent problems using a fire engine (urgent call) approach. For the first couple of months after my arrival,

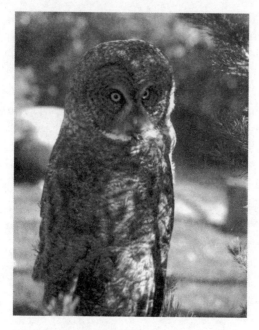

A great grey owl on its perch

most mornings we walked around the zoo, or I rode on the tractor with one of the keepers. Some days a slow amble around was just as rewarding. I had lots to learn.

In 1975 the concept of herd health—a look at the entire herd, rather than only worrying about individual animals—had been developing in veterinary medicine for several years. However, more often than not, the term herd health refers to pig production or dairy operations. The mix of species at the zoo meant that only the frame of the concept could work. I would have to create the bricks and mortar myself.

In addition to the vaccination program we initiated, there was the matter of diet. It was easy enough to see how the carnivores and birds were being fed, but when it came to the hoof stock, the feeding regime did not seem quite right. On my second Friday, as I sat on the trailer of the tractor driven by Jureen, I had a chance to see how it was done. He pulled up at each gate, and I hopped down and dealt with the gate as he drove into the pen and up to the side of the animal shelter. He scooped out several buckets of oats and filled a large wooden hopper bin. The animals obviously knew the drill as they began to amble over and stuck their heads into the trough below the bin. Jureen then cut the strings on several bales of alfalfa hay and dumped the feed into racks set next to the troughs.

Unfortunately, it was not really a good approach to dietary management for the variety of hoof stock we had in the collection. My best strategy was to keep mum about it for a short while to see how things unfolded. Making wholesale alterations all at once would not be diplomatic.

Throughout the days after my arrival I had of course been thinking of my family back in Holland. I had been staying at the Park Town hotel, which was nice enough, but 10 days was plenty and the university rules did not allow extended coverage for me.

One of my first non-veterinary contacts in Saskatoon had been with Dick and Jenny Neal, whom I had met in, of all places, a remote corner of Kenya's Meru National Park. It was my family's favourite park in Kenya and had the added advantage of only being a couple of hours from home. It was in that beautiful place that I had treated my first rhino.

She was the victim of a nasty bit of foreplay during which the bull had driven his horn up her rear end. The entire area had swollen so much that she had not been able to defecate or urinate for four days. She had stopped eating. An evacuation process—a 20-litre (4-gallon) enema—relieved the problem.

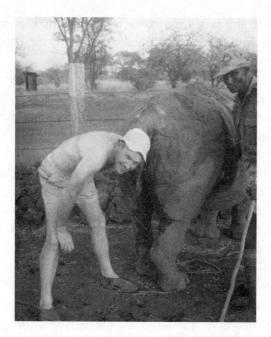

Not a selfie but part of a solution to severe constipation.

Dick Neal was on sabbatical studying reproduction in small mammals at the park, and we had shared cold drinks on the veranda of the house they had rented there. They at once suggested that we make contact as soon as we arrived in Canada. I met up with Dick on my third day in his office in the Department of Biology, just across the road from the vet school. He invited me to supper at their home.

When I told them that Jo was still in Holland, they at once offered to put us up when she arrived. They also mentioned one of their colleagues was about to leave for an extended working trip to Cuba. "You can take over our basement while you need it, and I'll ask Bruce and Carol if you can use their house when they leave. They will be away for about a month, so I hope that will give you enough time until you find something for yourselves," said Dick.

Fifteen days after my arrival in September 1975, I headed off to the airport with great excitement to greet my wife Jo and our children. It did not help that the plane was three hours late, and well past midnight when they appeared at the exit gate. The long flight from Amsterdam with the exhausted and cranky children—four-year-old Karen and three-month-old Charles—had not been ideal.

Not only was the flight late, but the airline managed to lose some luggage. Most of the lost items were not important. One item really mattered—Karen's favourite cuddly doll, a dog-like pink creation named Doddy that had long and much-sucked floppy ears. As if uprooting her from her home and pets (live ones) in Kenya and a trip around Europe were not enough, Air Canada had mislaid the one possession she valued above all else.

After much weeping and gnashing of teeth, and a sympathetic reception from the friendly staff at the luggage desk, we head off to Dick and Jenny's home. Doddy turned up in a taxi at three in the morning, having been found, along with other less essential luggage, in a corner of the airport. We quietly sneaked him into Karen's bedroom, where she had at last succumbed to the effects of the journey and tucked him in beside her. She sort of half woke, grasped him 'round the neck and with a small smile turned on her side, letting out a contented sigh.

For one of our first exploratory trips to the area we took the advice of several neighbours and colleagues and went to see the mountain that we had been told lay not far south of the city. We headed out on the highway and drove for 20 minutes, then onwards for another 20 minutes. Still no mountain.

Coming from Kenya, where you can see Mt. Kenya, the Aberdares or Kilimanjaro from great distances, well over 100 kilometres (60 miles) on clear days, we had expected to see something more than endless stretches of flat plain. As we drove past the small town of Dundurn, we did note a slagheap away to our left. It looked exactly like the slag heaps of the coalmines I saw during my student days all through the central rift valley of Scotland between Glasgow and Edinburgh. It even had what looked, from a distance, like some mechanical equipment of the sort that one sees on any kind of waste heap associated with mining.

Finally we reached the town of Hanley and realized that we had gone too far. There was only one thing for it. We stopped in at a gas station to ask about this "mountain."

"You passed it on the way, just east of Dundurn. It's called Mount Blackstrap," was the reply.

We backtracked and, feeling rather foolish, turned east at the Dundurn crossroads. The road soon dipped into a valley and crossed a causeway that divided a long, narrow lake. We had entered Blackstrap Provincial Park.

It was now plain that the mechanical equipment we had seen was a rather basic ski lift system snaking up from a wooden hut at the bottom of a slope near the lakeshore. The mountain consisted of an artificial pyramid made of garbage that had been added to the valley wall on the east side of the lake. Mount Blackstrap itself was built in 1969–70 for the 1971 Canada Winter Games that had been awarded to Saskatoon. The Mount Blackstrap website has more information: "The mountain covers seven acres [3 hectares] and has a 300-foot [91-metre] vertical rise. The length of the main run is 1400 feet [427 metres) and the length of the ski jump is 50 feet [50 metres]." The website also claims that the mountain "is a skier's haven and a training ground for many athletes."

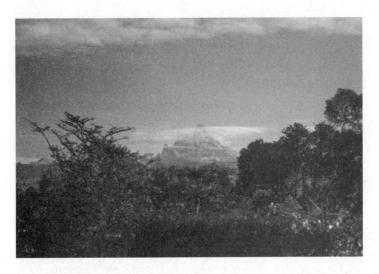

Mt. Kenya peaks through the trees

The "300 feet" was in *slight* contrast to the more than 3000 metre (10,000 foot) difference between our house in Nanyuki at 1975 metres (6480 feet), and Batian, Mt. Kenya's highest point, at 5199 metres (17,057 feet) that we could see every morning from our bedroom window.

Of course the Blackstrap website claims do not take into account the fact that the "mountain" has fallen on hard times. There has been no skiing there for a several years because nobody will take on the management.

Our neighbours and colleagues had a good laugh at our expense. We later found out that one of the nicknames for the human-made hill is "The Pimple on the Prairie."

Six weeks later we found a nice house, where we stayed for three years before moving to the countryside.

CHAPTER 4

Injections and Pedicures

The four members of the canine family at the zoo, coyotes, wolves, foxes and dingoes were obvious candidates for the distemper (also known as hard pad) vaccine. A badger and a pair of raccoons were the other resident carnivores that could succumb to this nasty disease.

They would all need two injections, six weeks apart, to protect them. In my student days in Glasgow enough cases of distemper in dogs appeared at the small animal clinic to make me wish never to see it again. Among the signs were hard footpads, a dry nose and an apparent cold. The disease affects the brain causing violent seizures, and death often follows.

It is all very well to decide to vaccinate, but vaccination requires handling, and handling implies close contact with the animals. This was not going to be a case of Mrs. Jones bringing Bubbles into the clinic in her handbag and plopping him onto an examination table.

I discussed this challenge with Brent as we tried to decide how to proceed. He needed no persuading and had a solution, at least a partial one. He reminded me of a tall cupboard in the large, old, yellow-painted, hip-roofed barn that stood out as a central feature of the zoo and a testament to the farming culture of the prairies. Even today these barns are still standing on many prairie farms. On any drive around the countryside one can see old ones, the paint long gone, tottering to one side and ready to collapse with the next storm. Those still alive are usually painted red.

In the zoo's barn was a collection of robust nets specifically designed for zoo work. Made of heavy nylon bite-proof mesh, they came in different sizes. Each had a drawstring near the top that, once pulled, would ensure an animal couldn't escape. We would be able to catch all but the wolves in the medium-sized nets, but the keepers would need a mixture of agility and bravery to do it. The team and Brent, either carrying one of the nets or ready to help, went into each of the enclosures. The animals circled around trying to avoid them. A keeper stuck out the net to snare the animal, quickly twisted it to prevent escape, pulled the drawstring and then stood on the neck of the net to keep it pressed to the ground. For the wolves, our team used the largest net, but even then the work required some guts. My task was then easy. The syringe slipped through the mesh, I quickly pushed on the handle once the needle was through the skin and the vaccine was in.

The raccoons and the badger were a different story altogether. They were housed in the barn, but the challenge in capturing the raccoons was their amazing agility. They can climb up almost anything, so the wire of the cage was no challenge. Once the net was over them, the animals had no trouble squeezing under its rim and slipping away to another corner of the enclosure. We finally managed it, but not without some interesting times.

The badger was easy to catch as he could not climb, but his snarling attitude was less than friendly. Had any of us been able to understand badgerian, or is that badgerish, his language would have been censored or bleeped on any media system.

I had no idea at the time that lions are also susceptible to this form of distemper. Indeed nobody did. It was not until the early 1990s that a dramatic outbreak of *canine* distemper occurred in the *lions* (hardly canines) of Tanzania's iconic Serengeti National Park. On March 2, 1994, Glasgow Professor Ray Holborn, happened to not only witness, but also record a short video of the violent convulsions caused by the virus in a Serengeti lion. It has been estimated that about a thousand lions, a third of the park's population, died in that outbreak.

The star attractions in Saskatoon were a pair of lions named George and Queenie. They needed a different vaccine, one against cat "flu." The disease is caused, not by a single virus, but by any one of four different agents or a mixture of some of them, and a flu virus is often involved. In domestic cats the virus can cause a variety of symptoms including those we think of when humans get the flu.

Obviously a net was not on the short list as a tool for vaccinating our two big cats. Big nets might have been okay for gladiators in the Roman forum, but the organizers of those events did not have to deal with the Office of Occupational Health And Safety. Moreover, where would we find a pool of spare gladiators should a lion emerge victorious?

The main problem was the design of George and Queenie's pen. With typically bright insight, it was Stu who came up with a way to vaccinate them. He mentioned that when he or his colleagues had to enter the pen for cleanup, they routinely enticed the cats away from the shelter by offering tidbits of meat through the chain link.

The next morning as Stu offered small pieces of meat to George and then Queenie, I stood next to him and tried to act like a visitor. The low outer fence did offer one advantage. I could lean over it. It was then simple to pop the syringe through the mesh and quickly depress the plunger. In both cases the cat's reaction was swift and angry, but the injections were in.

With the first round of vaccines out of the way, it was time to think of other pressing matters. As we walked around the grounds, Brent asked me, "Can we do something about the overgrown hooves on the sheep, especially the mouflons. They're pretty bad. As far as we know, they have never been trimmed."

"You're right," I replied. "One of the ewes and the big ram are in serious need of attention. Their hooves are so long that they curl up and over, almost touching their forelegs. But how are we going to catch them?"

"We can probably use the big cargo nets from the store," he replied.

It was then a question of planning. After coffee, the team and Brent went over the procedure. The entire crew was going to be needed for this operation because we would have to capture as many sheep as possible in one go, and then each animal would have to be held by a single person.

While waiting for the team to set the nets, I read the sign bolted to the chain link fence near the gate and learned that these attractive sheep, with their white saddles, dark brown and black hair coats, and the impressive sweeping horns of the males were of the Corsican variety. They were taken to the island perhaps as many as 3000 years ago from their original home range in Asia Minor.

Our plan was built around the fact that the shelters were not near the gates, which was, in this case, a boon. We could hook the heaviest net to one corner of the shed and lay the rest on the ground, with a rope attached at the other end snaking up over the fence. The end of the rope was to be pulled hard when the sheep got on the run and couldn't stop.

"We'll release the rope as soon as they hit the net and hope that it will collapse around them and entangle them," said Brent.

The entire procedure went like clockwork. The keepers went around one side of the building, and the sheep bolted. They shot round the corner and suddenly found

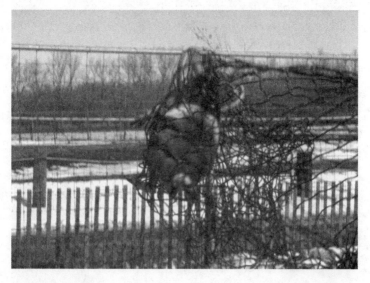

A high jump still means a catch

themselves going at full tilt into a net that instantly buckled and enveloped them. The ram made a spectacular jump as if to try and clear the obstacle, and I managed to press my camera shutter at exactly the right moment.

Obviously delighted with their success, the keepers each grabbed and hobbled a sheep with short ropes. Some "toenails" were badly in need of attention or had broken off. The younger ones, yearlings and lambs born that spring were fine.

As soon as we finished with each animal, it was released back into the grassy pen. Half an hour later the pedicures were done.

With the sheep hoof trims out of the way, at least until next year, it was time to boost the disease immunity of the carnivores with their follow-up vaccinations. To get a second dose into the now-wary lions, I rigged up a jab-stick that consisted of a sterile syringe on the end of broom handle. Once more Stu tempted them with treats, and

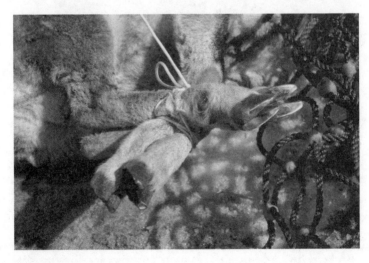

Hobbled legs

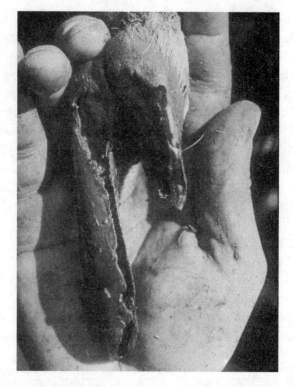

Twelve centimetres (4 inches) of overgrowth on one side only. The other has broken off.

I was able the finish my task. This was the last time that either cat let me get anywhere near them. The next morning they would have nothing to do with a proffered chunk of meat, and the pair moved away from me, snarling, with lips curled and neck hair erect.

For years afterwards, George and Queenie knew exactly who I was, even from distance. So much so that two years later, when I took the family to the zoo for a Sunday afternoon stroll, they recognized me from at least 27 metres (88 feet) away despite the fact that I was carrying our son Charles on my shoulders. I surely had a different profile and was now at least 30 centimetres (12 inches) taller, but I was still the nasty vet they knew and hated. The snarls were just as angry as before.

The negative reaction of the two lions, and other problems with the hoofed stock led me to consider another way to inject animals. It was a task I would have to do annually, not just to the lions but to other large creatures such as bison and the deer species in the zoo.

I could use the same gas-powered pistol that had worked on so many animals in Africa and that unfortunate first deer. I ruled that out for two reasons. First, it would involve putting a sterile vaccine into a compartment that could not be sterilized. Second, I had already seen that the explosive charge used to empty the pistol's chamber could inflict serious damage to the animal's tissues. This alone might compromise the whole endeavour and prevent absorption of the vaccines, rendering them useless.

I began to mull over ideas of how to achieve my objective, but nothing came immediately to mind. I let it stew in the hope that an idea would germinate.

CHAPTER 5

A Near Miss

I n the early days my job description not only included veterinary care at the zoo but also at the college for animals loosely classified as exotic. In the small animal clinic this basically meant anything other than dogs and cats. Birds, particularly birds of prey, were those most frequently needing my services. I had lot to learn, not just about the clinical part of the new challenge, but also the management of these special cases.

My clinical cases in Kenya had only involved one bird, a majestic sarus crane. Colleague Dr. Peter Holt and I had repaired a broken wing. The unusual part of the case was not so much the surgery as the location in which we did the work. It was in the sauna of the Mount Kenya Safari Club, where I had seen film stars David Niven, Michael Caine, Barbara Streisand and other famous figures. The manager had closed the bath for the day so that we could fix the broken wing with a metal pin.

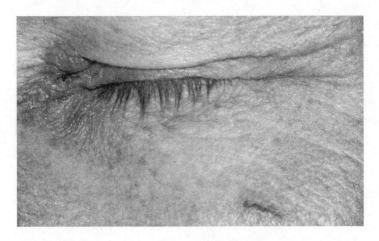

Talon marks top left on the lid and bottom right. A close call.

While viewing owls at the zoo was one thing, handling injured ones was quite another. The scariest moment occurred when I was still dealing with the unfamiliar. The patient, a snowy owl with a broken wing, was held in a birdcage in the exotic animal ward that also housed budgies, hamsters and a turtle while it recovered from surgery. Little did I know that owls can be aggressive. It was T.H. White in his book *The Once and Future King*, who described the raptor group as "birds of the foot." They need to be handled with the utmost caution.

As I leaned into the cage to grab him for a check-up, he leapt forward over my outstretched arm and attacked my face with his talons wide open as if he was trying to catch a mouse. He just missed a direct hit into my eye. It was only when the mirror showed how close he had been that I realized how lucky I was.

CHAPTER 6

Blowgun Development

I t is all very well to use a cargo net to capture mouflon sheep for a hoof trim and use nets for the handling of small carnivores no *bigger* than a wolf, but this equipment could not be used for anything larger or more flighty, such as white-tailed deer.

The seed of an idea about a new way to vaccinate the lions was slowly taking shape but needed more time to develop.

As we had to get on with the work, I began to use my dart gun, which also had its limitations. First, it was not very accurate. It might be fine when aiming at the broad expanse of the hind end of a moose or a rhino, and the difference between an actual aiming point and the hit was insignificant. It could even be used for elk and bison, but at a range of more than about 10 metres (33 feet) it was not accurate enough for the smaller and more delicate deer species and similar-sized animals. Moreover, it was unsafe to use on any animal that was not standing still. Any movement by the animal could easily cause the dart to penetrate the abdomen, thereby killing it. An x-ray of a small dog that had been darted in the belly by a dog-catcher made the point. The large dart, about the length of the animal's foreleg had penetrated the abdomen and killed the poor creature just as effectively as if it had been a bullet. There can be little doubt what the owners thought of that.

It was time to visit Barry Prentiss, the "Mr. Fix-it" expert at the zoo, to discuss a possible solution. We came up with an ancient idea from the European Middle Ages when castles were subject to occasional siege. Castles had many special narrow slits for use by archers. So Barry cut similar small apertures into each wall of the animal houses.

These worked well for a while, and I could take accurate shots at ranges from 5 to 10 metres (15 to 33 feet). The animals soon got wise to that method, and any movement or sound from inside an animal shed caused a spooked retreat.

Finally, an unfortunate event and a chance reading re-stimulated the seed of my darting idea. The incident occurred when the metal dart I regularly used emptied, as usual, in a fraction of a second into a deer's hind end. The dart contents, driven by a small explosive charge when the dart hit its target, plunged into the tissues. One deer died three days after being hit, and I needed to find out why.

On my arrival at the zoo, we had established the policy that any animal that died or was found dead on zoo grounds would be sent to the veterinary school for necropsy. In the post-mortem room, I witnessed a huge area filled with dark, clotted blood, about the size of a rugby ball in the muscles of the hind leg of the deer. The track of blood started just inside the point where the dart had hit.

It was obvious that the almost instantaneous driving force of the injection had acted like a bullet-driven needle. It must have cut through a blood vessel in the leg. I wondered what similar sort of damage I might have unknowingly done to other animals over the years.

In a serendipitous moment, while scanning the contents of a journal in the veterinary college library, a short article caught my eye. It was about the use of a blowpipe used to capture monkeys high in the canopy of jungles in Malaysia. Further research showed that blowguns or pipes have been widely used for hunting in many parts of the world, especially in South and Central America.

In all cases the tips of the darts were coated with a lethal compound (for the animal, but not for people who ate the meat). The resulting capture would be a tasty meal for the hunter. Another solution to the darting, especially the darting for vaccination, might be possible. The seed of the idea began to sprout. It seemed to me that we might be able to adapt the blowpipe idea for use in the administration of the vaccines and drugs.

The main challenge was to figure out a way of getting three to five ccs (about a teaspoonful) of drug into the dart and then having it empty into the target. Because I enjoy fiddling with problems like this in my workshop, after a few bouts of trial and error the solution came in a light-bulb moment.

Almost all syringes have a rubber plunger pushed by a handle that drives the drug into the patient. My idea was that we could substitute the handle with a second plunger placed just behind the first one and fill the space between the plungers with butane. To stop the second plunger from just shooting backwards as soon as the gas pressure was applied, I locked it in place with a needle broken off at both ends after being driven through the plastic and the

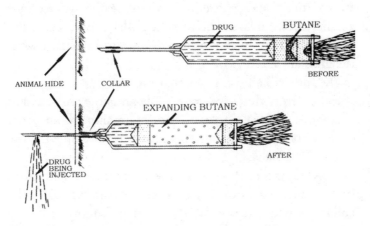

Top: The drug-filled blowdart just before it hits the target.
Bottom: The dart has almost emptied as the butane expands.

plunger. To allow the modified syringe to slide down a pipe, I cut off the flange at the back.

Then to the sharp end. The needle had to be sealed to stop the fluid from escaping until it was in the animal's body. A normal needle has an open tip, which would not work at all because as soon as the butane was inserted between the plungers the drug would shoot out. But dipping the tip into some epoxy glue dealt with that problem. The drug still needed to get out to do its job on the animal. A side hole seemed to be the best solution. At first I tried to make a hole with the smallest drill in my set. That was a failure. It made a hole so large it rendered the needle tip too fragile to withstand any kind of impact. Some tips broke clean off during the process.

A visit to a jeweller got me the kind of ultra fine bit that such craftspeople use. With the new bit held in a drill press, I was able to work accurately.

Next to test the system. When the new and improved needle hit a cardboard test sheet, it withstood impact. The next and final step in building the dart system was to place a collar over the lateral hole created with the drill bit. The collar would prevent any drug exit until it slid back against the animal's skin.

The other half of the equation was the pipe itself. Another visit, this time to a hardware store, solved that challenge. The dart fitted neatly into a thin plastic pipe. I filled the dart with water and pressurized it with the butane. No leaks.

Now to the test range in the basement. As the dart entered the target drawn on a stiff piece of cardboard, the collar pushed backwards. Presto! The butane instantly expanded, and the drug was administered into thin air against the workshop wall. No complaints, jumps or squeaks from the target. The seed had gone on to blossom. Success!

This first "blow" was successful with one limitation. As I emptied my lungs into the pipe, a significant volume of air escaped around the edges. The resultant noise was what one might call a tad rude in polite society, although kids laugh at the sound. Furthermore I realized that the loss of air around the mouth of the pipe would reduce the range of the device.

Back to the drawing board I went, again calling for workshop tools. This time I went to Barry's workshop at the zoo because I had no lathe at home. Barry recognized the problem at once. By noon he had created a wooden mouthpiece that he glued onto the pipe. No more embarrassing noises.

The finished product, 1.2 metres (4 feet) long, served me for the next 16 years. After some practice I could vaccinate or administer other drugs to a target 10 to 15 metres (33 to 50 feet) away and be sure of doing no harm, unless I was unfortunate enough to hit an eye.

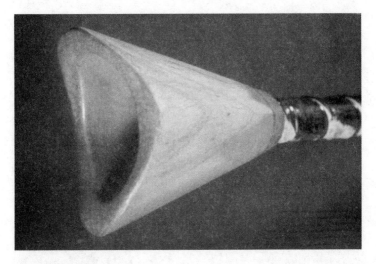

A wooden mouthpiece

Naturally I talked about the blow-dart development with colleagues, in particular Dr. Peter Cribb, head anesthesiologist at the college. Peter asked one question that I had not thought of: "Are you sure this thing is going to be legal and not classed as a restricted weapon?"

"I'm not planning to use it on anything other than animals." I replied.

"You might be wise to check," he said.

I did so with the RCMP, and they indicated the blowpipe would not be a problem as long as it was not used on people.

Thereafter George (the lion) received his yearly dose of flu vaccine. George did not seem to appreciate my efforts. Neither did he change his attitude toward me.

On a few occasions we needed to ambush him. I stood at one side of George's pen, blowgun in hand and raised into the "firing" position, while Stu stood on the other side, as innocent as a child who denies being naughty. While George's attention was focused on me, Stu pulled

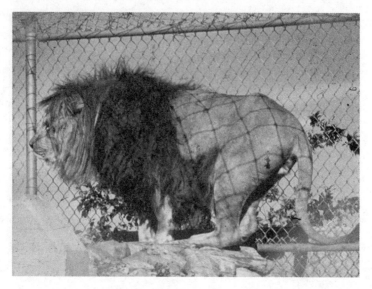

George reacts to his vaccination (left hip) by running up on top of the culvert.

another pipe from behind his back and administered the dose.

My duties as the zoo veterinarian covered more than just the animal collection. From time to time the blowgun proved invaluable in other situations. One such occasion was the result of a call from a worried homeowner who lived not far from the zoo grounds.

"There's a skunk in my swimming pool, and he can't get out. Can you help?" she said.

The striped (as opposed to the spotted) skunk is the main carrier of rabies in the prairies, so I approached the problem with great care. Stu and I headed to the house to see what we could do. When we arrived, we could see that the situation had an extra level of complexity. The skunk was not just in the pool. The bedraggled and soaking wet, thoroughly miserable, lump of black and white hair sat in the middle of the pool on the blue cover, the so-called blanket. Two glistening eyes, the only bright thing that identified the animal as more than a child's teddy bear, looked resignedly at us.

We went to the long edge of the oblong pool in the hopes of persuading the animal to escape at the other side. The skunk did shift away from us but only got to the pool's edge before we realized why it was using the centre of the blanket as a resting place. When it tried to reach out to the pool's edge, its weight promptly depressed the nylon material so that the skunk sank in the water up to its belly and could not reach the tiled rim. Carrying one of the zoo nets Stu quickly went to the other side, where the skunk was still trying its best to get out. It promptly retired to the middle.

The next possible solution was to use the blowgun. After loading the dart with a suitable drug cocktail, I went back to the long side of the pool so that the range would be minimal. The creature at once retreated. I could in no way ask my partner in this exercise to stand opposite me and drive the skunk back to the middle so that I could dart at a closer range. Such an action would be beyond danger-ous. The last thing either of us needed was for Stu to be darted if the projectile should ricochet off the blanket surface.

Back at the short end of the pool, the hours of practice paid off. The target was no wider than three of my palms held side by side. At a range of 15 metres (50 feet), I pinged the dart right into the skunk. Success! He was soon out cold. The housewife looked amazed, Stu seemed impressed and I was delighted. The rest was simple. I lifted the blan-ket's edge, causing the skunk slide down to the other side where Stu used the net to capture it. As a fisherman he had plenty of experience. Luckily the animal had not discharged its infamous scent, so we had no worries as we took it directly to the pathology unit at the vet school. I had no intention of doing a clinical workup and possibly exposing myself to rabies.

The skunk was not my only interesting encounter with urban wildlife. At other times there were stimulating white-tailed deer encounters in town. They both occurred in fall when young males are often driven off by big bucks wanting to ensure that any females became their sole (or is that soul?) mates. Under normal circumstances the young-sters head off into the countryside, but not always.

The first exciting event occurred when a buck leapt through the picture window of a house with a fine view of the university buildings across the South Saskatchewan River. Two ladies of a certain age were enjoying a quiet cup of tea when their afternoon view underwent a dramatic change.

The deer had no doubt come up from the bush-lined riverbank. Naturally it panicked when it found itself in the unfamiliar environment of a city sitting room. Soon shards of bone china mixed with the shattered glass of the window, and the ladies wisely retreated to call us. When I arrived about 15 minutes later, the room lacked what I assumed was its former pristine state. The sofa was shredded. The carpet was decorated with a fresh stain of something dark, wet and smelly. Several flowers lay scattered among greenery beside the coffee table.

A dart soon took the young buck down, and out it went into the zoo truck and away to a wooded spot well out of the city where I gave it an antidote. After 30 seconds it was up and away, without even a look back of thanks.

The following year the call came from another part of the city, well away from any bushes or other natural habi-tat. The deer had entered a small garden and proceeded to crash though a half-sized basement window. This time I was not alone. Someone in the family must have dialled 911 because when I arrived, two blue and white cars stood outside the house. A city fire engine was just leaving. I greeted the policemen as a visibly distraught young man told me about the invasion.

"It's in my room and has wrecked my guitar," he said.

The basement window gave me a clear shot as the deer stood shaking and petrified beside the single bed. Once it was down, we were able to get to the scene without difficulty via the stairs. The damage the deer had done was much worse than the ruined guitar. Both speakers linked

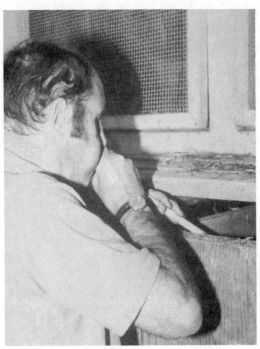

A shortened blowpipe in use for close-up work in a small pen

to an expensive sound system had been destroyed by repeated trampling of sharp hooves. I didn't know if there was any home insurance, but the lad himself surely took some time to recover from the experience. In the end, he also had quite a tale to tell.

The two burly policemen, who had obviously been fascinated by the unusual call, helped me carry the patient up the stairs and into the huge trunk of the Chevy. Twenty minutes later the deer bounded into the bushes just south of our home, 13 kilometres (8 miles) south of the city.

Currently, the most recent development in blowgun and dart development comes from Denmark. The dart has changed little from its second life when air in a longer chamber was substituted for the butane. However, the "pipe" has become a sophisticated rifle that uses CO_2 from an attached cylinder as the propellant. The range, up to 30 metres (98 feet), is calibrated by a pressure gauge mounted above the cylinder. The impact is no heavier than the blow dart. We used this "gun" extensively during the years that I took students to Uganda.

CHAPTER 7

Captive Bison and Farming

I had been in the city only five days when colleague Jim Smart asked me to come and help with some buffalo research. Jim is an acerbic, street-smart veterinarian whose professional reputation towers over his physical

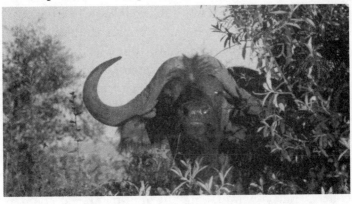

In Kenya's Nakuru National Park, a Cape buffalo gives me the once over.

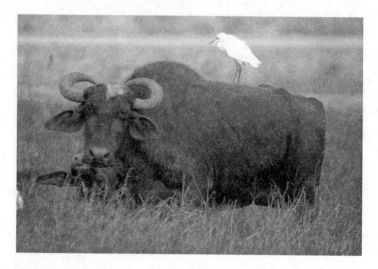

A water buffalo in Sri Lanka looks us over. His passenger is not concerned.

stature of 168 centimetres (5 feet 5 inches). I was not sure what Jim was talking about since the only buffalo of my acquaintance came from Africa or Asia. The African buffalo are the huge dark creatures that are reputed to kill more people every year than even lions.

The Asian ones are water buffalo. It soon became obvious that many folks, including veterinary students, get the Cape and water buffalos mixed up. But what I didn't know was that in Canada, the bison is often known as a buffalo.

I gave up getting my knickers in a knot about the name thing when a safari guide in India's state of Kerala called the massive gaur an Indian bison.

Curious about what was coming next, I clambered into Jim's grey Ford van, and we headed down the road. We were soon in the cattle yards a short distance north of the college. Tall, tough-looking but mild-mannered graduate student Alex Hawley was studying the dietary needs of

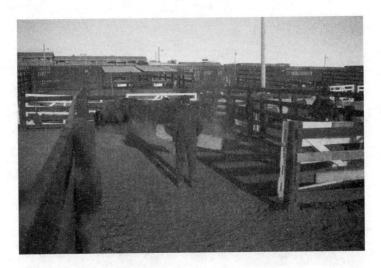

Alex Hawley, shield and bison

nine young males. My task was to collect blood samples from each animal once a month.

First we had to persuade them to enter the chutes. It was quickly obvious that they were not stupid. They circled round us, ignoring our shields. It wasn't clear whether the shields were intended to widen our profile or protect us. But with the four of us in action, the animals finally gave up and did what we asked of them.

These were not the only bison in Saskatoon. There was a small herd of a bull, four cows and their calves at the zoo. Of all the animals in the collection, they held pride of place for several reasons. They are huge, the bulls especially so, shaggy and very much an icon of the North American wildlife scene. They also hold an important place in the lives, beliefs and history of the First Nations people of the plains.

From the point of view of the zoo staff, and especially the zoo veterinarian, they have another quality. They need

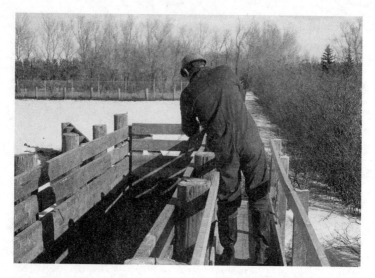

Blow-darting a bison

little in the way of medical intervention, vaccination once a year and a deworming if parasite eggs are found in the feces. Nothing more.

There are two important diseases for which vaccination is a must. One of these is blackleg, which, as its name implies, can cause horrific rotting muscle damage that almost inevitably leads to death. More important in terms of bison history is anthrax. Luckily a combined vaccine for both was available.

Anthrax, which had previously been reported in Wood Buffalo National Park does not just affect a few animals. If it breaks out, usually in wet years, it can be devastating, killing dozens or even hundreds of individuals. In the 1950s and '60s attempts at annual mass vaccinations had been made in the park, but so many animals were injured during the roundups that the idea was abandoned.

The treatments at the zoo were easy because the bison came to the set of robust wooden yards every day for their oats, and in later years more appropriate hoof stock pellets. When we closed the entry gate, the huge beasts had to go down an alleyway to the exit. Because they knew the way out, if we needed to work with them we could use a shield (a much bigger one than those used for research) to push them down the alley.

There they found their way was blocked with a stout barred gate. I stood on the elevated walkway to do what was needed. The vaccinations were done with the blowgun. Mostly this went well.

On one occasion, still remembered with laughter 35 years later by the keepers who were there, I fell into the corral when I leaned over too far to get at a calf. In the swirling dust I don't think the animals saw me. In any case, I promptly broke the world standing high jump record.

On the other hand, deworming was easy. Pouring the medication along their backs did the trick. No fuss, no muss, no worms after a couple of days.

The zoo animals could not go on the huge treks that their wild ancestors had done since who knows when; they lived in a 2-hectare (5-acre) pen. Therefore the normal wearing down of their hooves, a natural nail filing constantly applied when travelling long distances, did not occur.

By chance, because the bull needed a hoof trim sometime soon, I had the privilege of working on him with one of the giants of zoo animal medicine. At my request the eminent Professor Murray Fowler from the University of California at Davis came to the vet college to give a special seminar on zoo medicine. He was the first person to include this emerging discipline in a veterinary curriculum. Our students turned out in droves.

The day after his seminar, Dr. Fowler joined me at the zoo. Sharon Latour had just started as a volunteer and

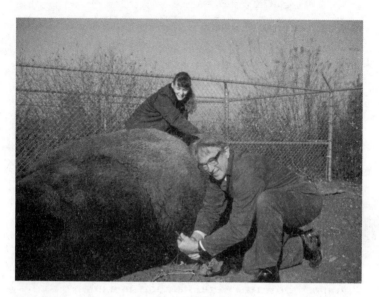

Dr. Fowler gets stuck in. Keeper Sharon Latour controls the bison's head.

happened to be assigned to hoof-stock duty. She was enthusiastic to join in the procedure.

A cocktail of drugs (not the same as for the skunk) worked best for immobilization of the hoof stock, and the drug-filled dart soon had the bull in a manageable state so that we could give him his pedicure. After the antidote injection, he was soon on his feet and grazing.

While the bison work could be planned ahead there was another occasion when we had to act promptly. One of the cow bison had had a losing encounter with a well-armed creature that probably weighed no more than one percent of the cow's 300 kilos (660 pounds). A porcupine had somehow clambered over the 2-metre (7-foot) page wire fence, or maybe under a gap at ground level, and the cow had been too inquisitive for her own good.

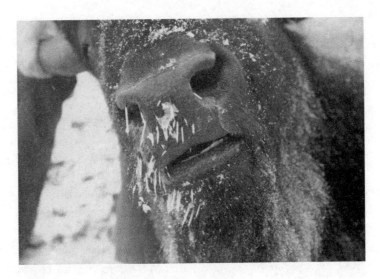

A bison's losing encounter with a porcupine

She ended up with a face full of quills, having chosen an inopportune time to mess with the original owner. Unfortunately, the wooden corrals were out of commission during a rebuilding so the immobilizing drugs had to be mixed up again. This time the treatment was all done and dusted in less than five minutes.

The surgical instrument used to remove the quills was neither sophisticated nor expensive. It was not even stainless steel, just a pair of pliers from the zoo workshop. A couple of dozen plucks completed the task. Then came a shot of antibiotic in case any of the quills carried bacteria, and finally the antidote.

There was one more serious occasion. One day the two keepers on hoof-stock duty asked me to take a look at the bull. Gerhard Steuwe, former deputy director of the Helsinki zoo before coming to Canada, was the senior of the two keepers. His experience with many species was often an asset. Tall, slim Perry Robinson with his Groucho Marx moustache was the other.

On their morning circuit they noticed that the big fellow was standing off by himself and didn't come up for his feed of pellets.

"There is something odd. He is uncomfortable," said Gerhard.

We took a look and decided that the stress of harassing him by a chase into the chutes might be the worst of two evils. Maybe he was just dealing with a gut ache from over-eating and would soon feel better. The next day it was obvious that he was even more uncomfortable.

The corral rebuild was complete, and we had persuaded the powers-that-be to invest in a new commercial chute system. This allowed us to easily get all the bison in, be examined, vaccinated and treated for worms without resort to the blowgun (or me falling in). Normally the saying about herding bison is that you can get them to go anywhere they want to. We had an extra advantage because the feed troughs and hayrack location had not changed. When the animals came in for a feed, the staff closed the entrance gate and the bison had to leave via the new exit.

We herded the entire group into the fancy new chute and let all the rest leave, which they did in a hurry. The bull followed but found the head gate shut. Generally a bison confined in this way objects in the only way he knows—he struggles and rattles the metal walls. This fellow rattled a bit, but with nowhere near his usual vigour.

During a standard head-to-toe workup (not actually as far as the toes) he seemed lethargic and was grunting more than normal.

"Guys," I said, "can you get one of the big poles that we used to use for a gate and bring it over?"

Perry went to the other side of the chute while Gerhard passed the pole under the patient's chest. At the count of three, they lifted sharply at both ends. The big animal let out a single loud grunt, not his normal "screw you" one, but in pain.

At veterinary college in Glasgow we learned that simple test for a condition called "hardware" that sometimes occurs in cattle. It is more properly called "traumatic reticulitis." The nickname derives from the fact that sometimes a ruminant will swallow a sharp object, often a wire or nail. If that happens the metal often carries forward and penetrates the wall of the misnamed first stomach (which is actually part of the rumen, the big fermentation chamber where grass is initially broken down by millions of microbes). If the metal object does penetrate, it will set up peritonitis and may even drive through the diaphragm into the chest cavity.

The situation needed a quick response. In my Kenya days, when I wasn't chasing rhino or stitching up a damaged lemur, I had dealt with cases of wire in dairy cattle by removing the offending object through an incision in the side of the grunting animal. A newer, easier, quicker and better approach is to simply feed the patient a magnet. Fortunately, just a short distance away at the college, the pharmacy had the special smooth, round-ended magnets, whose shape ensures that they can do no damage on the way down.

We also needed a long plastic, custom-designed probe with which to insert the magnet down the bull's throat. Meanwhile, the big bull waited, not very patiently, in the chute.

Eventually, we let him come forward through the head gate, but only as far as the crash gate 40 centimetres (15 inches) farther on. Without such a barrier, bison leave in a hurry before a handler has any chance of closing the head gate to grab the neck.

Then came the challenge. A bison can throw its head about with great force. Any attempt to get the probe into his mouth without restraining his head would lead to my arm being crushed between bison and metal. We restrained him even more with a rope tied to one side.

A bison's head is a lot longer than a cow's, and the probe had to reach past his tongue and into his throat where he would have no choice but to swallow the magnet. The only available probe was not long enough. The only solution was to jam a gag between the animal's upper and lower cheek teeth on one side and hope that he did not dislodge it quickly. If he did, those powerful teeth would turn my arm into man-burger.

First, we inserted the magnet into the recess in the forward end of the probe. Then with my naked arm, I shoved the probe as quickly as possible, pushing all the way up until I felt some resistance. I pushed the plunger, and the magnet did not fall out of his mouth. Thankfully, it had gone in the right direction down his esophagus.

Now it was a simple matter to give the bull a dose of long-lasting antibiotic and let him out to be with his mates, keeping an eye on him for several days. One of the best things about being a vet is to have successful outcomes to awkward cases. This was such a one.

A Small Fire Easily Doused

Some fires are more dangerous than others. Some can be put out with ease. This one didn't even need an extinguisher.

Mild-mannered, experienced Dr. Ken Armstrong, one of the team of field service clinicians, happened to bump into me as I headed out the door for my usual morning trip to the zoo. And I mean literally bump into…or maybe I bumped into him.

He was backing up as he talked to someone outside. I had turned to speak to Marie, our somewhat acerbic receptionist, as I headed out the clinic door. We turned and apologized simultaneously. Before going any further, he stopped and asked if I had time to go to the farm of one of his dairy clients, Mr. Sawatsky. He had just been there on an emergency call to deliver a calf that needed assistance to exit its mother.

While there, Mr. Sawatsky showed him a beaver that had somehow fallen into the manure-collecting trench behind the milking stalls. It could not get out because the deep, steep-sided trench had only a covered drain at one end as an exit. Ken's directions to the farm were straightforward.

Mr. Sawatsky was in the yard outside the dairy barn when I arrived. He was expecting me. We looked over the side of the trench. The beaver tried scrabbling up the trench wall, but then it headed to the other end, looking agitated.

"Have you got a sheet of plywood and some sort of slats?" I asked. We soon had the strips of wood, cannibalized from an old gate, nailed to the board about 30 centimetres (1 foot) apart. We slid the board into the trench as the beaver retired to the other end, as far away from us as he could get.

We moved away, and the animal went to the improvised ladder, ran up and vanished out the barn door. Job done.

CHAPTER 8

Helicopters at -20°

One never knows one's luck. The Haigh family motto is *Tyde What May*. In more modern terms this means "It will happen if it is going to."

I had been in Canada all of six weeks when Marie called from the reception desk.

"There is man down here who is looking for some drugs to capture moose. Can you come and help him?"

Talk about a stroke of luck. I had never seen a live moose, and this sounded too good to be true. I was down the stairs two at a time. The only new person in the reception area was a stocky bearded fellow. He was sitting on one of the pale blue upholstered wooden chairs looking at the board covered in overlapping posters advertising upcoming college lectures, a college bonspiel and two livestock shows.

We introduced ourselves. "I'm Bob Stewart," he said, "a biologist with the Department of Natural Resources.

We are planning to capture some moose for a research project, and I need some drugs."

He did not want to use a paralyzing drug that would immobilize the animals while they would remain fully aware of what was going on.

"That's not my way of doing things. I have heard of a drug called M99 that not only immobilizes but also renders the animal unconscious. Can you get some for me?" he asked.

I told him that this was not an option because M99 is a powerful form of narcotic at least a thousand times more potent than morphine. A veterinary licence is required to obtain any of this drug group, known as opioids, originally derived from opium.

Before he could voice his disappointment I said, "However, I have lots of experience with wildlife capture and am already using a similar drug at the zoo. So far it works well on deer. I'd bet it would do for moose."

"What does it cost?" he asked.

I told him that for a research project I could probably get some free samples from the manufacturer, based in Belgium, but that I also wanted to be involved in the work. He chose not to refuse my offer. After that the main question was timing.

I headed back to my office in a dream state. Dean Nielsen had told me that with my new position, I could write my own job description as long as the zoo work was done. This was a start—a true wildlife project. I looked forward to getting back to my favourite kind of work and a chance to learn more about my new home province. As it turned out, this "out-of-blue" call and the work that followed kept me excited and occupied from time-to-time in research programs with free-ranging wildlife for many years all over Canada and abroad.

By early December we were ready to go. The drugs had arrived. Our pharmacist, Fay Kernan, had ordered in some new metal darts and made up the imported powdered drugs into a usable solution. Bob's team was primed and keen. He called to fix the date. We packed collars and the tools we needed into black carrying boxes that looked like giant briefcases.

I remembered to load some duct tape into my own gear. It is the ideal stuff for holding many things together. One use, perhaps not mentioned elsewhere, is for taping a dart gun and a movie camera together to shoot footage as the dart is fired.

The other challenge was clothing. By late November it was colder than anything I had ever experienced. Luckily a store called Quinn the Eskimo carried used military clothing—mitts, parkas, proper boots with interchangeable felt liners—none of it I had ever seen before. But it was perfect.

In mid-December we loaded Bob's truck and headed north and east for four hours. He explained that we would be working on a big river delta.

"It's called the Cumberland Delta by just about everyone. It is really the Saskatchewan River Delta, but we will stick with Cumberland. Nobody will have a clue what we are talking about if we go fancy," he said.

Our base for the next 10 days was a trailer complex at Bainbridge Lodge. Here we met helicopter pilot Cliff Thompson and his light blue and white Jet Ranger. Eventually, he worked with us, winter and summer, for several seasons.

The trailer-turned-dining-area was next to my sleeping quarters, so a quick morning trip without the heavy gear was easy. Our hosts served excellent breakfasts—cereal, eggs and bacon with all the fixings, pancakes with their essential maple syrup topping, toast and marmalade. This early feed is a main meal for me, so that suited well. One definite downer: there was no kettle for making tea, and for me anyway, a tea bag dropped into a cup of hot water simply makes hot, brown water. Yuk!

My major concern for this research project was estimating the drug dose. A big moose weighs about the same as a big eland. But would practices used on the plains of Africa work on the frozen swamps of Saskatchewan?

The first moose, a male we darted in its hip, told me that the dose was pretty close. The animal, a good head taller than any of us but not as bulky as the eland, wandered about in a morphine-induced daze but would not lie down. A poorly thrown lariat that held only its nose solved that little problem. We were lucky that it held, but it was quite a grunt to pull him down.

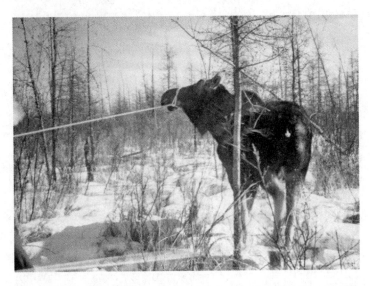

The moose is held with a rope around its snout. Note: It is a male with antlers recently lost.

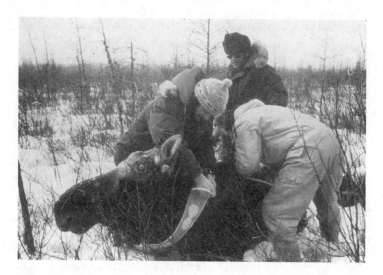

With collar fixed, we are nearly done.

We eventually developed a system that worked and managed to capture both adults and the young of the year. Bob was able to get more information about the status of his research subjects and, in a wider context, the province's population.

We had upped the drug dose by 20 percent, and the effect matched that of the moose's African counterpart. The animals would wander a bit and then fall down, which was all very well if the animals were in the open but it was more of a problem in thick bush where the chopper couldn't land.

From there I tried a technique that again came from Africa. It involved jumping out of the machine and catching up with the spaced-out moose, which was a singular advantage we had over any other species. A flap of skin called the bell hangs down from its throat, and when I grabbed it, I could lead the moose around like a large dog. Often Bob and I would join forces to pull an animal.

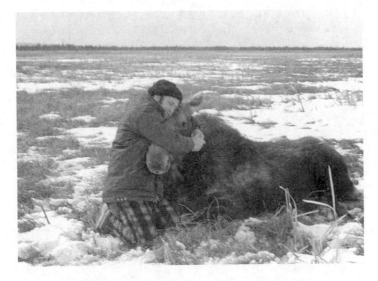

Taking a breather

After a walk through snow and the high rugby tackle, it was time to take a breather. My job, as the animal lay on the ground, was to check its health with stethoscope, thermometer and blood sampling. Bob and the team did their job with the collar.

The last measurement we took was weight. We built a sling with collar material, ropes and poles then hooked it up to a scale and lifted the animal under the chopper. Once finished, we gave the animal the antidote, and it was up and away in less than a minute.

Another *Tyde What May* event occurred in my second fall as a moose researcher. Bob mentioned that the North American Moose conference that year would take place in the city of Prince Albert, only a 90-minute drive north. The Super 8mm footage shot with the camera duct-taped to the dart gun generated considerable interest. Following the presentation, audience members asked several questions mostly about our moose-leading technique, which

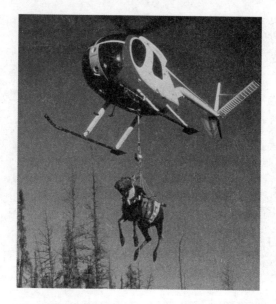

An unexpected lift

nobody had heard of or seen before. What followed were several invitations to join other teams. As a result, trips to a couple of projects in the neighbouring provinces of Alberta and Manitoba as well as Ontario let me spread my wings and learn more about my new country and the native moose population. Caribou also began to feature in our work.

Our contacts widened. The folks who organized the popular TV show *Mutual of Omaha's Wild Kingdom* called Bob a month later. We headed back to the delta to join the film crew the following November. Marlin Perkins, the show's white-haired host, came later to do the voice-overs.

Rod Allin was the main cameraman getting the dramatic shots of the chase and darting. With his round face almost covered in a dark blue hood he sat next to me in the chopper, but he was outside the machine in full body harness as we flew in sub-zero temperatures pursuing our quarry.

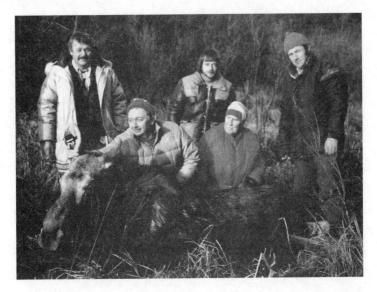

Wild Kingdom crew: left to right, Cliff Thompson, Ernie Jurgens, Bob Stewart, Marlin Perkins and author.

He must have been freezing with the wind whipping past him, but both he and slim, dark-haired Peter Drowne, second cameraman, got some great footage. The final title of the film was *Where Men Walk with Moose*. It is a delight to see this movie on YouTube 35 years after it was made. The fashion statement of long sideburns sets the date accurately.

My involvement with moose lasted more than 10 years and led to meetings with interesting people. Most remarkable among them was Antonin (Tony) Bubenik, who was fascinated by all things having to do with the deer family, in particular the role of antlers. As a talented artist, working mainly with watercolour crayons, he created a beautiful picture for me. It shows an event he witnessed when studying moose in the wilds of Ontario. A bull encounters

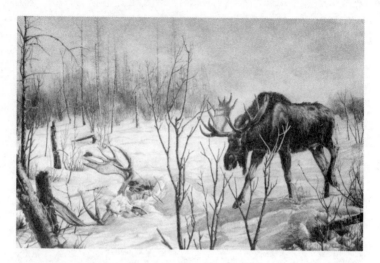

What on earth! Tony Bubenik's art.

a skull of one of his own kind with antlers still attached and does the moose equivalent of a double take.

I have been able to parlay Tony's studies and my own interest in the subject into successful storytelling gigs. The bottom line in antler confrontations related to breeding is that size does matter.

CHAPTER 9

Some Bear Facts

My first encounter with bears occurred at the zoo. In March 1976, I had been in Canada only six months and was just beginning to find my feet at the Forestry Farm Zoo, as it was called at the time, when two small cubs arrived courtesy of an officer from the Provincial Department of Natural Resources.

The two little cubs, weighing a little either side of 3 kilograms (6 pounds) (the male being the heavier), seemed fine. They had a good feed of evaporated milk, so Brent and keepers John and Jureen seemed happy enough to be left to get on with things.

As spring turned into summer, the cubs grew rapidly and were in an outside run by the time the school year neared its end. This seemed to be almost planned since many primary school class visits took place in late May when the weather was good enough for the students to be

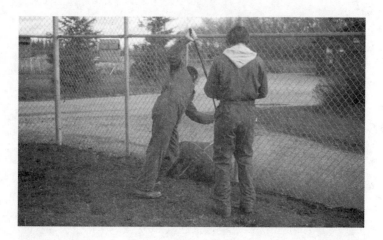

Bear in a net

outside, and the teachers wanted to take their students on field trips.

After three months the cubs began to lose hair over their shoulder areas, and Brent asked me to take a look at them. From outside the pen we couldn't diagnose the problem, so we asked the keepers on duty to help. It was not simply a case of walking over and calling the cubs to heel like trained dogs. These two growing guys would bite the hand that fed them, never mind mine. And so we decided to use the same heavy-duty nets that had worked well for vaccinating wolves.

In the end, the answer to the hair loss problem was simple. The door of the wooden house in their pen where they ate and slept had a rough entrance, and lots of hairs were caught up in the woodwork. The solution did not require medicine, but carpentry.

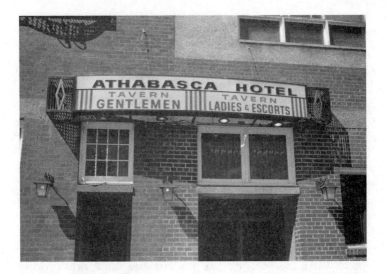

This sign is not exactly PC!

In our first June in Canada, after nine months on the prairies, we were suffering from a dearth of mountain scenery, Blackstrap Mountain notwithstanding, and decided on the advice of colleagues to take a summer holiday to Jasper. It was everything we had hoped for, and more, although not without a few surprises.

The first was the sign over the entrance to the Athabasca hotel. The outdated rule no longer applied, but the historic sign had been retained.

It smacked of the pubs in the Glasgow of my student days when women could not sit in the main rooms of public bars but had a tiny section, more or less cordoned off, where they could buy a drink.

The second surprise was the bears. I had not considered the possibility of an encounter, but the mounted board with its text and picture at the Mt. Kerkeslin campground, half an hour south of the town, made it clear that we should be extra careful.

The first sign by the entrance was quite clear about the common-sense rules:

"When Camping, Be Aware! You Are In Bear Country!"

There followed a list of 11 things to never leave unattended at a campsite. The feature items were anything to do with food as well as toiletries and garbage.

A young, blond warden in his mid- to late 20s, who introduced himself as John Steel, came by soon after we set up our tents and warned us about a problem bear in the area. John was dressed in the standard pale brown uniform and wide-brimmed hat, and he reinforced the sign's words, adding that the tent would be no deterrent. A bear would simply rip it open if he smelled anything interesting. For us it was a case of déjà vu. Exactly the same precautions have to be taken in Africa with the major campground pest, the baboon.

The solution for keeping the baboons at bay was rather easy. As long as a campground attendant patrolled the area swirling a slingshot in his hand, the monkeys stayed well away. We had seen the result when a baboon ignored the man. A stone would soar out of the sling as if fired from a gun, and if the shot was on target, which it usually was, the monkey would depart in haste. Watching the attendant swirling his ancient weapon and practicing on innocent rocks reminded me of the Biblical tale of David and Goliath. However, in Canada either nobody had thought of the idea or could not imagine paying an attendant to patrol each campground. Regardless, no such service was available, so we had to take extra care with our goods and chattels.

John Steel and I were soon on the subject of problem bears and their habit of returning to the same campground time and again once they had found out that the place was a potential source of grub. From there we moved on to capture drugs, and I told him of my successes with other carnivores. He suggested a visit with the chief warden might lead to something useful. Another good reason for the visit to town was the need to purchase a fishing licence.

John's suggestion yielded encouraging results because the warden service, like others, was struggling to find a good capture drug for dealing with problem bears. They could be caught in culvert traps, but then the only recourse was to hitch the trap to a half-ton and haul it away to somewhere with road access to release it. Some bears needed to be taken farther into the backcountry, hopefully far enough from human contact to prevent their return.

The chief suggested that I return the following summer, bringing some drugs with me to see if we could find a solution. He even suggested that there might be some funds available for the work.

I am more of a catch-and-eat rather than a catch-and-release fisherman, so my new licence and the rental of a rowboat on Moab Lake proved ideal. An evening rise of rainbow trout attracted by a home-tied size 16 Royal Coachman gave us an excellent supper. Many years later, on a wonderful trip to Canada's Yukon, I learned that the Dene people of the region feel much the same way; they believe to catch a fish and the return it to the water dishonours the fish.

Back at home it was time to get on with the zoo work, but the Jasper experience stayed with me. I began to research information about drugs that had been used on bears in the past. The Google and App generation wouldn't realize that in the 1970s the only way to do this kind of research was to go to a library and start digging into books and journals. The vet college library was well stocked so it didn't take me long to find what I was looking for.

The first drug had been a muscle relaxant called succinylcholine, "sux" for short, which had a narrow safety margin between inadequate, effective and lethal doses. In one study carried out during the mid-1960s, almost half the black bears immobilized with this drug had needed artificial respiration just to keep them alive. Another unpleasant property is that sux only paralyzes a patient; it does not remove any awareness. The animal may be unable to move, but throughout any handling period it is aware of everything around it, which is not exactly a welfare-friendly situation. There are a few records of humans injected with succinylcholine for sound medical reasons when the real anesthetics did not work. These subjects were terrified by the paralysis and by the fact they could do nothing at all to alert the doctor.

In bears the recovery stage was also quite unpredictable. One minute the bear seemed to be out cold, and the next it would be up and angry. Given the fierce reputation of bears, sux was surely not a drug to instil confidence in a researcher.

Then came PCP, whose proper name is a 26-letter alphabet soup—phenylcyclohexylpiperidine. It is more commonly known as phencyclidine or mercifully even further shortened to PCP. Even a few drops, 4 to 8 milligrams, causes hallucinations in people. PCP was and still is an illegal recreational street drug. The term "recreational" hardly seems to fit the accounts I've read about the drug, which were more like horror stories. One young man tore his own eyes out under the influence. In another report, a man threw himself down an elevator shaft because he thought he could fly. The stuff has more than 20 street names, Angel Dust, Rocket Fuel and Embalming Fluid among them. One researcher found that PCP induces symptoms in humans that are indistinguishable from schizophrenia.

In humans a dose of as little as one milligram can cause strange behaviour. Effects in people may last from four to eight hours when the drug is used recreationally, with after effects lasting a day or two. Each "cc" contains 100 milligrams, and one would certainly not want to accidentally inject oneself or even splash a drop or two into one's eyes or mouth. Considering the evidence of effects in humans, there is no way of knowing what sorts of hallucinations animals have suffered on being subjected to this drug.

The two zoo bears had grown into large and dangerous terrors by the fall, and we did not have the facilities to care for them. Since they were to be shipped off to another institution in a few days, I decided to test a morphine-like drug called fentanyl, which is about 100 times more potent than morphine. Of late, fentanyl has been in the news because addicts have not understood its potency. Several deaths have been associated with its use, especially when sold by unscrupulous drug dealers.

In Canada the drug had only been used on humans, dogs, moose and mice. I had used it extensively in Africa on all sorts of creatures, from elephants and rhinos to a variety of antelopes and dogs because it has the great advantage of being quickly reversible with an antidote.

Over the years, when I had to be knocked out for a surgical procedure, I have enjoyed joking with my anesthesiologists about the fact that I was using fentanyl on rhinos at about the same time as it became part of the arsenal for human pain relief and preparation for full anesthesia. It also became the drug of choice for open-heart surgery.

The drug worked a treat. After my limited trial in the fall on the two zoo bears it seemed to be a safer drug than the others written up in the journals. It was worth a try for

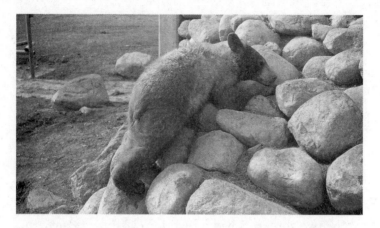

Falling asleep on fentanyl. The hair loss over the shoulders is visible.

the Jasper animals, so I wrote a small grant proposal for only $200.00 and sent it off to Jasper. It was quickly approved, and with that letter, came a request to give a couple of workshops, one in Jasper and another in neighbouring Banff National Park.

In Banff, we tested the drug on grizzly bears with the same success as at the zoo. In this case we didn't get out of the vehicle but fired from the safety of the warden's truck.

During the next summer it was no hardship to go back to Jasper for further testing of the fentanyl. Rather than camping we booked into cabins in town. Jo's sister Gerda joined us, and so the five of us set off in late June for another mountain fix (not to mention fishing).

The work and the workshop went very well; we immobilized and transferred half a dozen problem bears. Two of them had been caught in culvert traps and were sedated so that they could be put into a sling and helicopter-lifted far into the backcountry.

The blowgun was ideal for our purposes. From a range of only 1 metre (3 feet) or so from the grill of a culvert trap a miss was hardy possible. The lightweight plastic dart

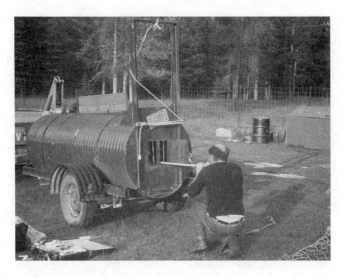

An easy shot into a culvert trap

would inject the bears without the risk of hurting them. This is in stark contrast to the heavy metal darts that had been the standard almost everywhere in the world for 20 years.

We had some interesting challenges when working with other wardens in campgrounds with nuisance bears. In all but one case I could not use the blowgun because we could not get within the 10-metre (30-foot) range limit beyond which a miss would be more-or-less a certainty. At greater distances the dart gun, which offered a sure shot up to 27 metres (89 feet), was the main tool. But then I also had to make sure that no gawking tourists and campers were in line with the gun when I had the opportunity to take a shot. In the end, we got some good exercise chasing those bears after the darts hit home, and they took off into the bushes.

By a strange coincidence one of those bears was spending time at Kerkeslin, where we camped the previous year.

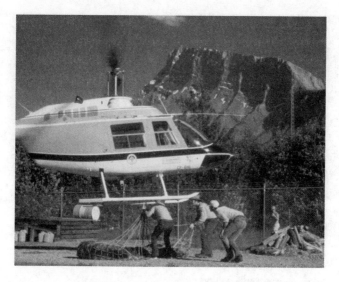

A drugged female bear and her cubs are ready for lift-off.

He was a recidivist and had been moved out twice before by road. This time he was airlifted over two mountain peaks, beyond Mt. Edith Cavell to a spot near the Amethyst Lakes on the park's western border. We thought that the job might finally be done. Not so. John Steel told me the next day that the bear had found its way back to Kerkeslin by the following morning! Unfortunately, in the 1970s, problem bears got three chances and then they were out. Later the park service folks found a better way of dealing with these problem bears. It began in the campgrounds with the installation of bear-proof garbage bins.

Before we left Jasper that year, we had a memorable fishing evening on a midsummer night. Jo and I sat in a rowboat on Patricia Lake above the town, while Gerda did the childcare duties at the cabins. The evening sun dipped behind the mountains, but plenty of light shone in the sky at 11:00 PM when I shipped my oars and pulled the cork on a bottle of Chablis that we had chilled ahead of time in

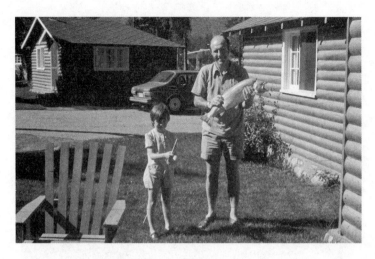

Karen is not impressed, but she is only six.

the cabin fridge. The plastic "glass" was just about to touch my lips when the reel on the fly rod started to scream. A nearby American tourist came to help with his big net, and 15 minutes later we had a nice fat rainbow in the boat. The American had had no luck all evening, so I passed him the Mrs. Simpson streamer that had attracted our catch. I could easily tie another. It was too late to get an official weight, but on my little scale the fish registered more than 5 kilograms (10 pounds)!

CHAPTER 10

A Canoe Trip
with a Bonus

The success of my trials with the fentanyl for bear work at the zoo and in the mountain parks was tempered by the discussions I'd had with the wardens in Prince Albert National Park, which is three hours north of Saskatoon.

We have spent many camping holidays and overnight stays in this beautiful part of Saskatchewan over the last 40 years. It all began with a canoe trip above some rapids on a small river in the park when Charles, not yet a year, went on his first boat ride. He was more-or-less blocked by tents and other gear and told to sit very still. We were on our way to Kingsmere Lake for a camping-cum fishing trip. As a dedicated fisherman, I naturally took my rods and other tackle along.

There was a narrow-gauge rail line on the way to the lake. It was built because the shallow rapids down to Lake Waskesiu were impassable. The line had been built for

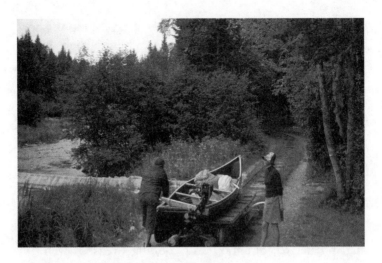

Heading back from Kingsmere on the tracks

transport of powerboats, but we took advantage of it with our canoe as had countless others.

To get to the railhead from the parking lot, I portaged our canoe on my shoulders for a short distance. As we all walked along, I chatted with a kindred soul as keen on fishing as I was. His name was Paul Galbraith, a park warden, but he was not dressed in the brown uniform and wide-brimmed hat of his day job. He was off duty, just heading up to the lake for some R&R.

We chose a site at the campground aptly if unimaginatively called South End. Our au pair Celia, who had joined our family from England, was with us on her first-ever camping trip, and Jo and I decided to test our skill on the more open waters of the lake. We had not heard of the lake's fearsome reputation for sudden squalls, but we soon learned.

Luckily I had spent a good deal of time messing about in boats as a lad and knew enough to get us out of trouble before the wind really got going, but we had to crab across the lake as the sudden waves threatened to swamp the boat if we stayed on our current heading. Had I been on my own in the canoe, I would not have been able to manage. We ended up on the lee shore a long way from our tents.

Back at the campsite we had a scary surprise. Celia told us that soon after we had set off, a bear had wandered into camp. He started by tearing off the door of the outhouse. He no doubt failed to find what he was looking for, so his last port of call had been the table where some of our gear had been placed. We had read enough about the danger of bears and food to ensure that not a single edible item lay within easy reach, not in the tents, nor on the table. We had hoisted all our food and cooking utensils, even our toiletries, into a nearby spruce tree after enclosing it in a hay net and slinging a rope and pulley over a high branch. We had not reckoned on the curiosity of bears.

Our uninvited guest had seen the 20-litre (4-gallon) clear plastic water jug on the table and climbed up to investigate. As Celia put it, "He tried to push it a bit and then he put one foot on top and pressed down. The jug burst, and the water sprayed in his face. He jumped off the table and ran off."

On the way home I dropped into the park headquarters and found Paul ready to check on a nuisance bear report. He told me that he and his colleagues had to deal with as many as a dozen such events in any given summer, and that our water-bomb story, while funny, likely involved a bear known to be a problem at the South End campsite. It did not take long to convince him that I might have something new to try as a suitable drug mixture for bear capture if the animals could not be lured into the dark green culvert traps that were duplicates of the ones used in Jasper and Banff.

I had come to realize that there was no way that vets would be able to get to all the bear capture events that occur every summer across the country. While my trials with the morphine-like fentanyl that had proved to be effective in the mountains were encouraging and scientifically interesting, the strategy was not practical for non-vets. As park wardens in either national or provincial parks, these folks had special skills. They also needed to drug bears from time to time, but a veterinary licence was needed to use opioids, as this class of drugs is known. This was not an option.

Luckily I had been testing a variety of drug combinations to try and improve safety for both humans and my animal patients since the late 1960s during my time in Africa. It was an alternative for bears that the wardens would probably be able to use as long as they had some training and a permit from the government minister. It had worked well on cats of many sizes, from domestic tabbies to leopards and lions and seemed worth a try. I ran the idea past Paul, and he and his boss agreed that we could give it a go. I then just had to wait for a call, which came sooner that expected.

In less than a week I was struggling out of bed at 6:00 AM, making a quick cup of tea and gulping down a bowl of cereal more or less at the same time as I struggled into trousers and a sweater. Two and half hours later I was loading my blowgun before peering through the grille in the trap door and puffed the first-ever dart filled with the new mixture of drugs into a bear. The combination worked like a charm. Five minutes later he was out. Of course, we prodded and poked him to ensure he was not going to wake up, but it seemed as if we were off to a good start.

Naturally I did all the standard clinical checking and was delighted to find that everything was normal. Steady breathing, strong regular heartbeat, no change in temperature over the next 60 minutes. When the bear began to show signs of waking up, we loaded him back into the trap. To release him, I joined Paul and one of his colleagues, and we headed off to a remote corner on the western edge of the park. A bonus for me was to learn that Paul and I shared a passion for fly-fishing. I have been accused of having 10 percent heron genes. If that is true, then Paul and I share a common avian ancestor somewhere back in the mists of time.

That passion translated into an invitation to try one of the stocked lakes, not far from where we dropped off the now fully awake bear, and we spent an absolutely soaked half-day trying our luck. Not a fish showed any interest in any of the several flies on offer, but I learned a new and invaluable field-craft skill. To get some relief from the downpour we stood under a thick spruce tree as the rain hammered down on the lake, making pockmarks as big as saucers, when Paul suggested making a fire. I watched in amazement as he pulled a length of soaking wet and rotting birch bark from an old, fallen stump, shook it a few times to get rid of the soggy interior and then held up a cigarette lighter to one edge. It took a while, but the bark flared and we had the makings of a fire. The fire burned for quite some time as we piled on more of the same and reached up for some slightly less soaked twigs from the spruce trees nearby. I'm not sure that the little fire actually warmed us, but it was certainly a morale booster. I have used this handy skill many times since, and of course, most outdoorsy Canadians have known it all along. I suspect they learned it from the original inhabitants of the land. Nowadays I consider birch bark to be a basic piece of camping equipment.

By the time I had made half a dozen more early morning trips to Waskesiu, we were sure that the new mixture was both safe and effective. We had even gone to the park dump a couple of times and captured adult females with cubs so we had a range of weights on record. The only thing left to establish was the maximum safe dose for a bear so that wardens need not worry too much about the difficulty of estimating the weight of a bear in a trap.

We took our kids, Karen who was seven and Charles three, on another camping trip to Kingsmere. This time there were no wind problems. We made an early start from South End, and our next stop was at the Pease Point campsite for a bite and a brew. As we glided to towards the shore we saw something that made us change our minds. And quite by chance I had my Super 8mm camera with me.

We watched a successful fisherman place a stringer of fish on the nearby cleaning table and turn away, presumably to collect his filleting knife or some other item he had forgotten. As the man disappeared through the willows toward the campsite proper, a medium-sized bear emerged from the bushes and grabbed a single northern pike. I checked the camera-on switch and pressed the trigger. The bear was only 10 metres (33 feet) from us, and I recorded his climb and turn as he headed back the way he had come, no doubt ready for a midday feast. Of course the rest of the fish, still attached to the chain, followed suit. I did not wait to record the fisherman's return to the table and can only imagine his reaction. Puzzlement, for sure. The rest of the scene lies only in my imagination. That short length of footage sits gathering dust among too many little blue canisters of film somewhere in our basement. It will no doubt end up in the trash in the not-too-distant future.

Beyond the table, as the channel to the next lake in the chain narrows, a beaver lodge stood right by the water. As we sat on the top with a glass of juice and a sandwich, a cow moose emerged from the willows opposite. Just behind her came a single light brown calf. The pair of them walked through the rushes by the shore and headed straight towards us. It was only when they swam to a spot about 10 metres (33 feet) from us that I woke from my moose-induced trance. I stood up, making some noise. Mother moose turned sharply, entered the rushes on our side of the water and headed away into the spruce trees. Unfortunately, my camera was still in the canoe.

The last bear we processed at Waskesiu was well known to the wardens. He was a serious problem animal, raiding garbage cans, scaring children and being a general nuisance. An outdoor barbeque on the deck of a cabin might well mean an abandoned meal and steaks for the bear. Despite his repeated transfer to remote areas of the park, he homed in on the townsite like a racing pigeon.

He had created havoc one too many times in the campgrounds and summer cottages right next to the community, and he was undoubtedly trap-happy. We had tested the new mixture on as many bears as possible, but this was our chance to test the effects of an overdose as the nuisance bear was to be shot. The animal was resting comfortably in his green tunnel. My blowgun did its usual job as I knocked him out with a standard dose, which gave us one more data point. Once we had weighed him in a net slung under a tripod, I drew up a large syringe and added more drug, up to six times the dose we knew worked well. The large volume would not fit into a dart, so Paul and his colleagues weighed him under a tripod so that I could be sure of an accurate volume of drug.

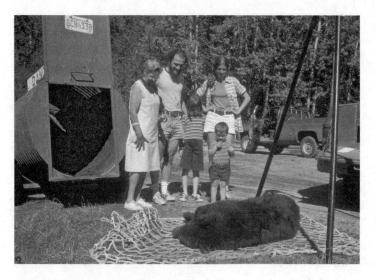

Family and friends from Kenya look on.

We loaded him back into the trap and waited…and waited. Three hours later the bear had not moved, except for his slow, steady breathing. My family, who were with me at the time, wandered off for goodies at a local donut shop. Paul and I took quick separate breaks for some refreshment. Then it was back to my vigil at the trap.

Eventually, six hours after we first darted him, the bear started to move a bit, lifting his head and twitching his tongue in and out. Thirty minutes later he was sitting in the trap, looking less than pleased, and I had my answer on safety.

CHAPTER 11

Hippo Dentistry

My most unusual case did not come from Saskatoon. One day, I received a called from Greg Tarry. At once, in my mind's eye I saw a dark-haired, slim man who towered over my 182-centimetre (6-foot) frame.

"This is Greg Tarry from the Calgary Zoo. Don't know if you remember me." We had worked together on an elk that we brought to the zoo from Banff National Park. An unknown person had killed the zoo's resident elk with a crossbow.

"What can I do for you?" I asked.

"We have a problem. Our hippo, Foggy, needs some attention and we do not have a vet at the moment. His upper and lower canine teeth on the left don't meet properly. When he chews they are not wearing each other down as they should. The upper one grows out sideways so the lower continues to grow upwards. It is now so long that it cuts into the inside of his upper lip. He has quit eating. He can't even close his mouth properly. He is obviously in pain, and we think the tooth needs cutting off. Of course we can't do that without sedating him. Can you get here and see if you can do anything, please?"

Fortunately, I was able to book a seat on the morning flight to Calgary. Then I headed to the well-stocked vet college library, put on my thinking cap about the "how to" and dug into the scientific literature to see what I could find. The results were not encouraging. Three reports mentioned a variety of drugs, but all cautioned that the hippo is difficult to deal with.

I didn't work with them in my Kenya days but knew instinctively that they should not be sedated while they are in water because they are likely to drown as the drugs take effect. The references confirmed my intuition. One source even mentioned driving a road grader into the water then using the blade to push the patient out onto dry land before it became fully immobilized. Another suggested the use of fentanyl. Because I had used it so often on other species and someone had previously used it on a hippo without fatal results, it seemed worth a try. Another advantage was that the college pharmacy had it in stock. Foggy weighed half as much again as my former rhino patients, so I calculated the dose accordingly. I also took into account another piece of advice from my sources: using long needles is essential when sedating hippos.

Alas, none of the researchers mentioned anything about teeth in their studies. That would prove to be as interesting as the drug selection issue. Dealing with extraction never entered my head. Pulling Foggy's tooth would not be a walk in the park.

After an uneventful flight to Calgary, I found myself with Greg as we looked over a high wall at the hippo.

He had been locked out of his pool and was standing quietly in a passage between his daytime (water pool) and nighttime quarters. Hippos in zoos must have a water pool to be comfortable and well cared for. Foggy was mouthing but not munching on some lettuce. A stout steel gate confined him at either end of the passage. My first worry had been allayed. The patient was not going to be able to get into water until we deemed it safe.

We descended and went to the front of Foggy's pen to look into his mouth. Even a flashlight didn't help. It was not possible to get a good look, as he did not appear to want to open up. Trying to persuade him was not an option, but the keepers assured me that he needed help. His left canine tooth was embedded in his upper lip.

Hippos have a fearsome reputation for aggression. When East Africa was home, Jo and I had often, in many parts of the continent, watched them submerge, surface, snort, fight and generally carry on.

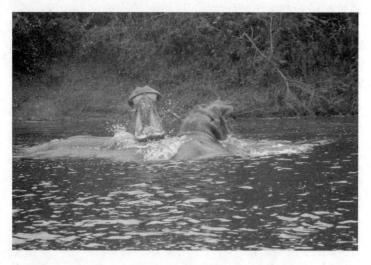

Two bulls duke it out in Uganda's Lake Mburo National Park.

We saw our clearest example of hippo aggression as we paddled on the Zambezi River in Zambia. Before we set out, Christmas, our whiplash-thin guide, admonished us to follow him carefully to avoid the home territory of a well-known, bad-tempered bull. To emphasize just how bad-tempered the hippo was, Christmas took us past a canoe lying on the bank that did not exactly look sound. Two jagged holes, each more than half a metre (almost 2 feet) long, had been ripped through the hull on one side.

"One of my guests did not listen to me and went too close to a bull we know is bad," he said. "The bull came up out of the water and bit the canoe. The man was very lucky. The teeth went through the boat and missed his leg, which was between those two big teeth." We did not need a second warning. That image remains clear even without the photo.

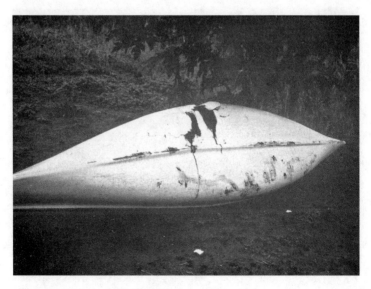

After an encounter with a bull hippo

Foggy needed sedation, but my blowgun system failed. The dart simply bounced off as if his hide it were a tractor tire. Sticking an arm through the cage bars to administer a hand-held injection was not a consideration.

Back to the drawing board. Finally, I rigged up a syringe with a 10-centimetre (4-inch) needle at its business end and attached it to the end of a broom handle. With duct tape to hold it in position, I climbed up above the passage to get a bird's eye view of Foggy. With a single thrust, I pushed the jab stick directly into the back of his neck, just right of centre. Five minutes later Foggy obligingly dropped to his haunches close to the stout bars. It took only a moment to lift his lip and see the problem. Every time he tried to bite down, his lower tooth would drive into the gum above it. Poor fellow. It must have been painful. No wonder he was off his food.

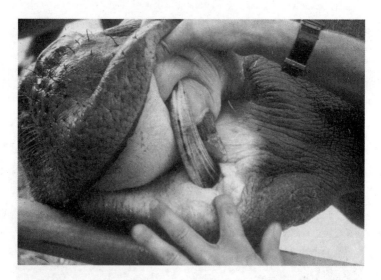

Foggy had pronounced overgrowth because the teeth did not wear each other down.

Because the bull was still somewhat aggressive, we waited another 10 minutes before I set to work. He was still not fully anaesthetized but was sufficiently sedated that we could proceed, as long as we got a rope onto his head to control him. All seemed well, so the keeper filled another big syringe with penicillin and stuck it into his shoulder.

Unfortunately, angle grinders had yet not been invented. If they had, it would have taken only a few short moments to chop off the top bit of the offending tooth. In this case a saw was our only option. In anticipation of the task, I had packed a flexible wire called a Gigli saw, used by veterinarians all over the world for emergency obstetrical work to cut up a dead calf that is stuck in a cow's body.

The Gigli saw was named after its inventor, Italian obstetrician Leonardo Gigli, to make bone cutting easy. British secret agents carried the Gigli saw during World War II. Its main feature is a rough surface, a bit like a coarse file, that allows it to cut through bone quickly and efficiently, a great asset when doing field amputations of any sort.

Dr. Gigli had surely never tried to amputate a hippo tooth with his invention, and I only just managed it. The entire role of wire, all 3 metres (10 feet) of it, was just enough. The problem was that after only a few back-and-forth strokes, the wire broke, right in the middle, of course, where it had been grinding on the tooth. This left two short useless pieces impossible to hold. I quickly discovered that hippo tooth is the hardest substance I had ever worked on. Forty years later, I've not found any other harder.

Eventually, by using ever-shorter pieces of wire and holding the ends in my hands rather than attaching them to the saw's handles, which required extra lengths to do so, I was able to get the job done. It took almost an hour to complete the task, by which time my hands were raw from the rough treatment.

All the while, I kept an eye on Foggy's breathing to ensure that my anesthesia was working properly. I did not want him to wake up prematurely or perhaps not wake up ever again. One of Greg's staff helped by calling out the breathing rate and writing it in the medical record at regular intervals. I was greatly relieved because the scientific articles in the vet college library had not filled me with enormous confidence because none of them indicated a sucessful outcome.

With the tooth work finally completed, Foggy needed an antidote to wake him. I was worried because the scientific articles stated that veins are difficult to find because of all the fat layers in a hippo's body. Fortunately, either luck or instinct kicked in because the first place I tested was his foreleg, just below the bend of his elbow. That is the spot where nurses and doctors, whether of humans or animals, have drawn blood from millions of patients. I found a nice fat vein, as big around as a ballpoint pen. I don't know where my predecessors had been looking because it was an easy hit.

A minute after the antidote began to circulate in Foggy's body, he was standing and seemed none the worse for wear. Still, we agreed to keep him out of his pool overnight. I headed home on the evening flight.

After this event keeper Mona Keith of Calgary took the wise step of training Foggy to come to the cage bars to trade treats—lettuce and other favourite foods—for good behaviour. This enabled her, and keepers at other zoos, to spend a few minutes every day gently grinding down any incisor that threatened to create the same problem—surely a more elegant and risk-free approach than waiting for another crisis to occur.

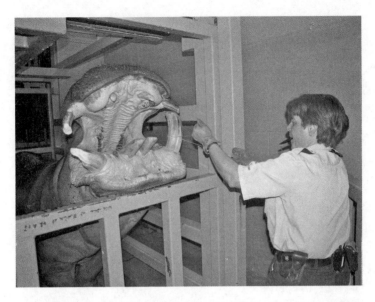

Mona Keith trained Foggy to allow her to cut his lower tooth. The upper abnormal one is growing sideways.

While working with Foggy, I was reminded of my Kenya years. Hippos are fascinating creatures. They emerge from waterways in the early evening to graze, sometimes advancing a long way from the rivers or lakes in which they spent their days. Occasionally they will graze during daylight hours, but they always return to the water. Like many other water-dwelling mammals, hippos are thought to have been land or semi-aquatic creatures for millions of years. In this regard they share a common trait with whales, to which they are distantly related, although hippos have not gone as far down that reverse track as those wonderful creatures have.

The scientific explanation for the long-term history of the semi-aquatic life of hippos is modern. There is, however, an old folktale that provides a different explanation for the hippo's need for an aquatic habitat:

According to the East African story, hippos did indeed once live on land but were constantly burned by the tropical sun. The suffering hippos went to their king, Kiboko [kiboko is the Swahili word for hippo] *and asked him to speak to the great god Ngai, who live on top of the snow-capped mountains. They sought permission to live in the water.*

Ngai replied, "Never. If I allow that, my poor little fishes will all perish because you will destroy them and eat them up with those great teeth of yours."

So, the animals remained on land, but when the hot season returned, they again suffered terribly. Indeed, their skin was burning up and turning red. They went back to Kiboko and pleaded with him to ask the god Ngai once more for permission.

After thinking for a long while, Ngai granted the request, but under four conditions.

"First," he said, "you must only spend the day in the water. At night you must leave and go on to the land. Second, you must never again eat any kind of meat, but only eat grass. Third, when you return to the water in the morning you must shake your tail when you do your business so that I can check to see that there are no fish bones in your dung. Finally, you must open your mouths very wide from time to time when you are in the water so that I can check to see that there is no meat stuck in your teeth."

Jo and I have told this story to hundreds of school children and adults in Kenya, Uganda and even Canada and the U.S. With the word poop substituted in the right place, the story gets a laugh from any audience.

The taxonomic name for the subspecies of hippo that occurs in East Africa is *Hippopotamus amphibius kiboko*. The scientist who chose the name was surely paying homage to the name used by the people who lived among the animals.

The red hue on the hippo's skin is not sunburn but rather one of two naturally occurring pigments that not only have a sunscreen effect but inhibit the growth of disease-causing bacteria.

Hippos do indeed eat only grass, but tail shaking is a behaviour males use to mark their territory. Their big incisors are not used for eating; the other teeth do that task. Instead, the incisors are used for threat displays and fighting, especially among males vying for dominance in pods. When a hippos opens its mouth wide, it is actually showing off its large incisors as a warning.

When it comes to snow-capped mountains, there are three possibilities for Ngai's home in this story: Mount Kilimanjaro, the highest African mountain; Mount Kenya, which we were fortunate enough to be able to see daily from our bedroom window and the Ruwenzori Range, also known as the Mountains of the Moon, that straddle the Uganda—Democratic Republic of Congo border.

Foggy lived on until 2010, having had several dental procedures. The zoo staff took the reluctant but humane step of euthanatizing him because his advanced arthritis no longer responded to treatment. He was 47 years old when he died.

The Loneliness of the Long Distance Owl

The engineer of the freight train must have been surprised when an owl smacked into his front viewing window as he guided his vehicle west out of Winnipeg. Luckily the window was large enough that the bird did not obscure his vision. The unlikely collision occurred only 20 minutes after the train left Manitoba's capital, so the owl remained stuck in the recess for the best part of 10 hours on the way to Saskatoon.

By 2:00 PM the injured great horned owl was on the examination table in front of me. The bird was in trouble. Both wings were broken, and his beak was smashed.

We'd had several cases of vehicle–bird collision previously. Many could be repaired but not usually well enough to fly and find food, but they were fine to become teaching examples in schools. Some could even be rehabilitated in the flight cage beside the clinic. This owl had no chance of a decent life. We made the decision to end its pain with a lethal injection.

A happier outcome was the case of an owl with a broken leg. An X-ray was scheduled to determine how bad the break was and whether we could fix it. The x-ray image was a surprise. The bird had actually been shot. The leg had three pellets in it, one of which had hit the middle and split the bone. The repair was relatively easy for my colleague and experienced surgeon Dr. Steve Withrow. I ran the anesthesia while he inserted pins and placed a cast around the leg to hold everything together.

A month later the cast was off, and afterwards he went out to the flight pen where he was exercised daily to help him regain the strength he had lost while sitting in his cage. I took him to our home a few days later. He sat on a fence post for a short time before flying off.

Owls, and other raptors such as red-tailed hawks, are often brought to the to the vet school clinic by well-meaning

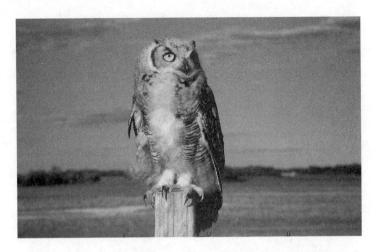

A brief look round before heading off across the prairie landscape

members of the public, most having been injured by vehicle impact. Some can never be helped and are euthanatized. A few, such as my owl patient, can be released to the wild after being exercised in flight pens.

A small number become useful as teaching aids and are taken to schools by volunteer members of the zoo society. The star member of that fraternity was a Swainson's hawk. She was found in a field by a local farmer when she was just a fluffy ball of down, likely having fallen out of her nest. After a few weeks at the vet college, where she was cared for as her feathers grew, the zoo society took her over. They named her Ariel. She lived for 23 years. As Lesley Avant, a long-time member of the society told me, every school kid in the city must have met her at least once.

CHAPTER 12

The Graveyard of the Atlantic

The beauty of working as a half-time zoo veterinarian is that it gave me free rein to pursue the free-ranging wildlife side of my university post.

The first was the amazing opportunity to get involved in moose research with Bob Stewart and his team. The next followed soon after. The call from a man identifying himself as Dr. Harry Rowsell at first confused me. He quickly put me at ease by telling me that he had been a member of our own faculty as a pathologist and was now working at the medical school in the nation's capital in the same capacity. He named several of my colleagues and referred to my interest in wildlife. From there he quickly segued into an interesting pitch.

"I am the current chair of the Canadian Council on Animal Welfare. This year I am also the chair of the Committee on Seals and Sealing, handily known as COSS, while the actual chair is on sabbatical."

Of course I was at once interested, if a little puzzled as to the reason for the call.

He went on. "Would you be free to join me and Mr. Tom Hughes from the Ontario SPCA on a trip to Sable Island to find out how we can help with some seal research?"

You can no doubt imagine my enthusiastic reply, although I did warn Dr. Rowsell that I had no experience with seals. I did not tell him that I had hardly ever seen one never mind that I had no idea where Sable Island was located.

Basically the winter grounds of the hooded seal were unknown, and the COSS folks wanted to find out more about their ecology and lives in order to protect them. It was known that they pupped and bred in spring in the Gulf of St. Lawrence, but where they got to after that was a complete mystery at the time.

The plan, as Dr. Rowsell outlined, was to go to Sable Island and test systems on the grey seals that have their pups on the sandy beaches there. If we could develop a good technique with the grey seals, then we could apply it to the hooded seals. The critical factor was the date for our trip. It had to take place during the short period between Christmas and early February when the seals would be on land. They would either be about to pup, feeding a newborn or breeding. As soon as the pups were weaned and the males had done their thing, the seals would be back out at sea feeding on fish.

The narrow window had everything to do with the remarkable growth of the pups. They weigh about 15 kilograms (30 pounds) at birth, and for the next three or four weeks they add weight at a furious rate as they suckle five or six time a day for up to 10 minutes at a time. The milk is rich in fat, so that by the time they are hardly more than a month old, they will have at least tripled their weight! And as soon as the pups are weaned, the adults get on with propagating the next generation.

We all met at the Toronto airport, and I had a chance to get to know Harry a little better. He was one of the most charming and gentlemanly people I have ever met, and we shared a common interest in many things related to the environment and conservation. Tom Hughes was a bluff Yorkshireman, and we also shared a common link. My parents had lived near the city of York for four years after my dad retired from the Highland Light Infantry and learned the ropes as a salesman for King George IV whisky, a Distillers Company Ltd product. My first summer job as an 18-year-old had been in a pork pie factory right opposite the Rowntree's chocolate headquarters on the northern edge of that city.

We stayed overnight in Halifax and then headed to the airport to board a three-engine plane known as the Trislander to get to Sable Island. Strangely, on that model, the engines are not where you'd expect them to be. There is one on each wing, but the third is near the rear on a rocket-like projection just in front of the tail. The "island" part of the plane's name refers to the Isle of Wight off England's south coast. My amazement took me back many years in a flash to family connections. Both of my grandmothers had lived on the IoW for many years. Granny Haigh returned there after her husband, my naval captain grandpa, died. She purchased Lee Farm and so was near her Ball family siblings, who were successful business folks. My grandparents on the Wall side of the family moved to the town of Cowes where granddad, a naval architect and naval engineer (a rare combination) lived out the last 10 years of his life. The two grannies resided half an hour apart by road, but when I was a lad that was too far to go on the island's narrow twisting roads for just one meal. It had to be lunch and tea or tea and supper. The Trislander was developed in the town of Ventnor on the island's southern coast, an hour's drive from either granny!

The pilot explained that the advantage of the Trislander over the other aircraft was that the plane could both land and take off in a short distance. This was a good thing because Sable Island did not have an airstrip, and we would have to put down on its northern beach at low tide. This gave us a narrow window for arrival. We had almost 300 kilometres (190 miles) to go, and conversation, other than at high volume, was not really an option. I drifted off into a snooze and woke as we began our descent.

I was too late to take a photo of the whole island, which seemed to stretch in a long, lazy curve a long way to the east. The island is about 42 kilometres (26 miles) long, but less than 1.5 kilometres (1 mile) wide at its widest point.

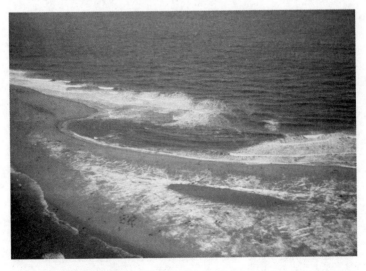

Near the western end of Sable Island. The black dots on the left are seals.

Beneath me all I could see was a stretch of sand dotted with what looked like seals.

As soon as we had gathered our luggage from the belly of the plane, the pilot did a quick 180 and taxied back along the damp sand toward the other end of the beach where he made the same quick turn. With a roar, the plane accelerated from almost stationary to full throttle. It leapt into the air like a fly escaping from a futile attempt at a swat and headed westwards.

A taciturn elderly staff member with a scraggly mop of white hair and a face wrinkled by wind and age picked us up from the beach. He drove us a short distance in a battered and rusting old Ford half-ton truck to the main station. The "road" was simply parallel ruts in the sand bracketed by coarse grass browned in its winter dormancy. He explained that the island had been continuously occupied since 1801 and was now principally a government weather station. Part of his attitude was probably due to the fact that he was one of the last people to have been born on the island. He seemed to resent our presence and did not like what he may have seen coming in the way of a tourist invasion. We stopped at a white clapboard house that was in need of a coat of paint.

Sable Island only became a National Park in 2013, 35 years after my visit. Before that it had been a rescue station for mariners (and still is), a coast guard station and it also had the dubious distinction of having two lighthouses, one at each end of its long crescent. Not surprisingly, its other name is "The Graveyard of the Atlantic." Since it has witnessed at least 350 shipwrecks, the name is well earned.

One consequence of the many wrecks, especially those in the days of the sailing ships was the establishment of a thriving population of horses. We had arrived at midday and couldn't get to work right away so the chance for a late

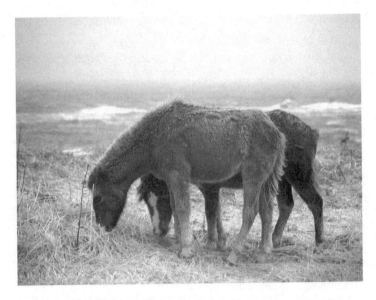

Tough, dry winter-feed for Sable Island ponies

afternoon walk over the dunes was enticing. The first thing that struck me was the icy wind coming off the Atlantic. The vegetation was nothing more than the same tough-looking grass on which ponies were grazing. Widely separated single sticks of dead-looking shrubs stood like miniature flagpoles.

The descendants of those hardy horses dotted the landscape in small mobs. Whatever they had looked like when they left Europe, they were now ponies, all fairly uniform in size and colour from dark to light brown.

With the pony processions along the beach, close encounters were typical. They had no fear of people. In late February, their heavy winter coats made them look scruffy—warm and windproof was the state of affairs as the winter gales swept in from the open ocean.

The next morning, after a hearty dose of porridge and a strong brew, we headed out west for no more than

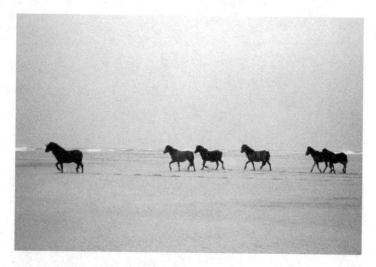

Pony procession on the beach

a 10-minute walk to the beach where we could see a couple of dozen seals lying around.

We tried at first to catch one in a net, but he was too much for us and soon thrashed his way out of the mesh and headed off, in high dudgeon no doubt, to the shore, where he vanished into the waves. As we knew that hooded seals, our real objective for the research, were both larger and more aggressive than these rather placid creatures, we moved to the next level—the dart gun. In the absence of any other information, it seemed worthwhile to once again try my favourite immobilizer, fentanyl.

It was an interesting and pleasant change to have no worries about a moving target. The only thing I did to make sure of success was to adapt the short commercially available needles that had worked for Foggy the hippo. The hippo's thick layer of fat under the skin was similar to that of the seals. The drug needed to reach the muscles, and it would be ineffective if it ended up in the fat. I'd had a similar challenge in Africa with building needles for

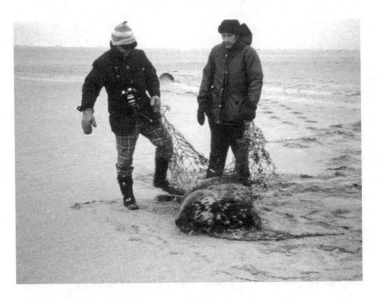

A grey seal soon wriggles its way out of the net.

rhino work. In that case the need had been to penetrate tough thick hide.

The work went smoothly but with one big and scary surprise. The seals stopped breathing within three minutes of being darted. Completely. They were not dead; their hearts beat regularly, but the breathing stoppage was unexpected. No marine mammal, nor indeed any lung breather, can breathe under water. The natural solution when a whale or seal dives is the so-called dive reflex. Breathing at once ceases when they submerge, and the oxygen-rich blood supply is diverted to the brain and heart. Any intake of the outside water (as opposed to air) would mean death by drowning. The drug had somehow caused that same dive response.

There are a few high profile news stories about very young children surviving after falling into cold water. The speculation is that they experience the same dive reflex and

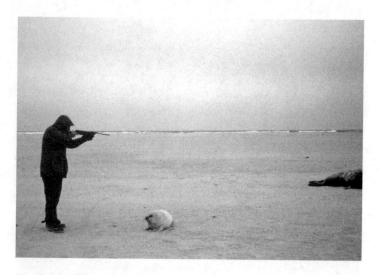

The female offers an easy target. Her pup, lying a short distance away, simply looks at the intruder.

become like aquatic animals. It is not clear if it is the age of the children or the water temperature, but several children have survived for many minutes. It is certain that the parents don't think about the finer points of cardiac physiology as they hug their little ones after such an incident.

When the seals went into their own dive reflexes because of the drug action, we were not concerned about a long period of immobilization, just the ability to make it happen. Seals have a huge vein that runs along their backs, so it was easy to inject the fentanyl antidote into the bloodstream and satisfying to watch them regain consciousness within 30 seconds.

We did not confine ourselves to live seals and could not stop looking at everything around us. Several logs had washed up on the beach along with old bits of rusted metal, likely debris of a wrecked ship. They stood at random spots like gravestones in a bombed-out cemetery. We saw a few dead pups on the beach and naturally,

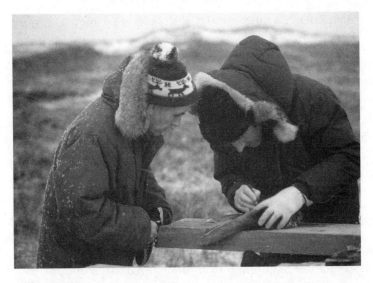

Dr. Rowsell, at left, looks on as I probe the rear flippers of a dead pup to try and learn more about its death.

as a pathologist, Dr. Rowsell wanted to find out more about their demise. It was no problem to put their bodies onto the flat surface of an unidentifiable structure for examination.

After examining three of the pups, he concluded that that they had most likely starved. They may have been abandoned when their mothers went out to sea to feed and were taken by Greenland sharks. Or their mothers had left or lost their milk because of harassment. The brief pupping and breeding season is mayhem with non-stop sounds of females moaning and howling as they try to protect their pups. In addition, the sound of dozens of bulls making low-frequency grunts has been described as being similar to a steam train. The males constantly fight for breeding rights. They not only bite and tear at each other, but also at the females that object to their advances.

Inexperienced mothers may simply have escaped to a more peaceful place.

In the end we found so many live seals that we were able to finish up our work in two days and head home. Harry was obviously satisfied with our results because within the week he was back on the phone to Saskatoon asking *how soon* I could be free to travel to the gulf of St. Lawrence to carryout the next phase of the study.

In the present day, a massive change in the ecology on Sable Island since the '70s has resulted in the grey seal population ballooning from the estimated 12,000 in 1977 to roughly 242,000 in 2007. More recent data are not available. Part of the reason for the increase is likely the disappearance of large predatory fish such as the Atlantic cod because of overfishing coupled with an increase in smaller fish (including young cod), the seals food source.

CHAPTER 13

Hooded Seals

D r. Rowsell called to confirm the flights, and I was again off to the Gulf of St. Lawrence. Harry told me that we would be based in the town of Grindstone, or in French, Cap-aux-Meules, on the Magdalen Islands.

I soon found the islands in the atlas and was intrigued by the long narrow shape and multitude of small islands that make up the group. How we would get there was one question. They lie 80 kilometres (50 miles) north and east of Prince Edward Island, and some 150 kilometres (62 miles) west of Newfoundland and a tad farther from the eastern tip of Quebec's Gaspé peninsula. The islands are politically part of *La Belle Province* so another name for them is *Les Iles de la Madeleine*. Like Sable Island, this island group has been the site of hundreds of shipwrecks. The residents there are the French-speaking descendants of 17th century French colonists.

For this trip, a young graduate student, Pierre-Yves Daoust, joined the team. Pierre-Yves had obtained his veterinary degree in St. Hyacinth veterinary college, which is part of the University of Montréal. He is fluently bi-lingual, which proved to be an asset.

Pierre-Yves and I set off in early March. After a long, convoluted series of flights in ever-smaller aircraft via Halifax and Charlottetown, we arrived late in the evening of March 16 on the islands, and were met by biologist Robert Stewart from the University of Guelph and technician Wayne King, who would be working a third season in the gulf.

We had only a narrow window to work because by the end of the month almost all the hooded seal pups would not only have been born, but with the shortest known lactation period of any mammal—a mere four days—be fully weaned. This is because the females produce milk that is up to 60 percent fat. Once lactation is complete,

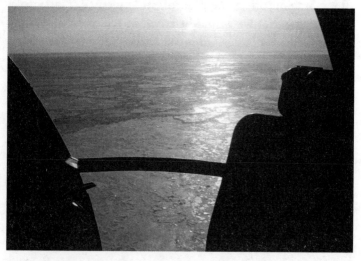

Ice on the gulf viewed from the helicopter

the females get back to breeding and by early April no seals remain on the ice, even if any big enough patches persist by that time.

Our helicopter pilot turned up in his bright yellow machine the next morning, and we headed east of the islands across vast expanses of pack ice.

In 1978 when our team did its study, the ice pack stretched for miles. In 2014 Pierre-Yves told me that the ice situation is now a problem for harp seals during the whelping season because for several years the ice conditions have been poor.

Other than the fact that we were to work on seals there were few similarities between this trip and my work on Sable Island the previous month. For starters, the seals were more widely scattered across the seascape. Second, we were on ice the whole time, and Rob warned me not to get too close to the animals. They could move a lot faster on the slippery surface than any human, and the males

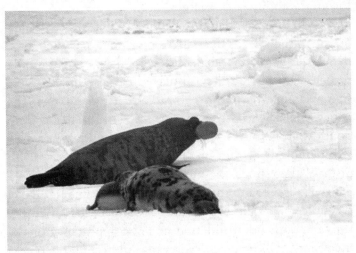

A bull and female hooded seal close together. The bull's hood is inflated.

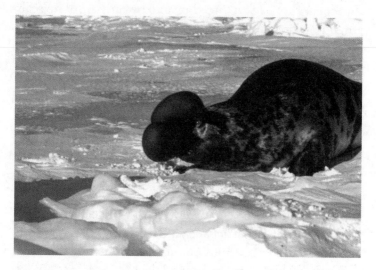

Hood inflated as Rob gets near (© Rob Stewart)

are known to be aggressive. Third, at up to 400 kilos (900 pounds), the males were almost twice the weight of the grey seals on Sable Island.

Fourth, the males had big flabby bladder-like structures on top of their heads that sagged down between their eyes, hence the name "hooded." That hood was not the only sexual characteristic they displayed because finally, there was a fascinating surprise for Pierre-Yves and me. The males, especially those in attendance with females, and no doubt waiting for the chance to breed, would evert a dark red membrane of thin material from their left nostrils in display. They shook the membrane up and down as they emitted a low roar. From the sac came a rattling noise like a couple of garden peas rattling around inside an empty tin can. Both hood inflation and the appearance of the membrane indicated aggression toward us interlopers.

Our task was to tag the hind flippers of as many seals as possible because the knowledge of where this particular

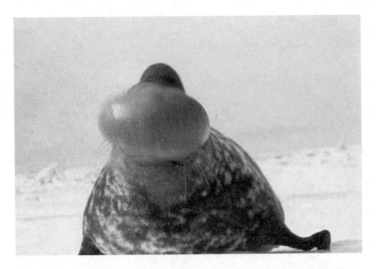

The sac is fully extended. This guy means business. (© Rob Stewart)

breeding population spent their summers had either been lost or was never known. A population of hooded seals had recently been observed on pupping grounds in Davis Strait between Baffin Island and Greenland, and another question about this colony near the Magdalens was whether the two were connected.

Regrettably, we were working 30 years before satellite-linked radio tags that allow for long-distance tracking were developed. This meant that the best available technology was to put a plastic tag into each hind flipper of as many animals as possible and hope that someone would report seeing them in a different place.

With the valuable experience of the Sable Island work under my belt and the doses of fentanyl bumped up accordingly, we were soon able to work as an efficient team. It took between three and eight minutes for the drug to take effect in females, and slightly longer in males. We were careful approaching all the animals, and I soon

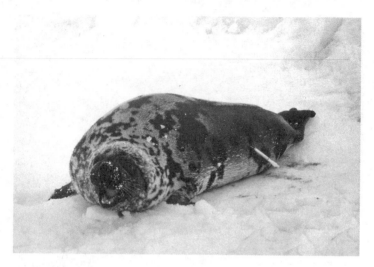

A darted female

realized that I had to fire the darts from farther away than I had planned. Females with pups nearby lifted their heads from the surface and began to curl back their lips to give us the evil eye if we got any closer than 5 metres (15 feet).

Even after darting, we took precautions using a long rod that Rob had brought along, reaching out near each seal's head to see if it was safe to proceed. As I tested the dose, in some cases I needed to top the animal up to make her safe to work with.

The tagging process took much less time than the wait for the drugs to work. All but two of the seals received a fast-acting antidote within five minutes, and while most stayed put, the four animals that moved away actually returned to be near their pups within two-and-half minutes of the injection. We also brought along a net, thinking it might allow us to snare a seal, but it proved useless even in a partially drugged female that tried to get away.

Half of the females we injected stopped breathing altogether. Although I knew hooded seals can dive for up to

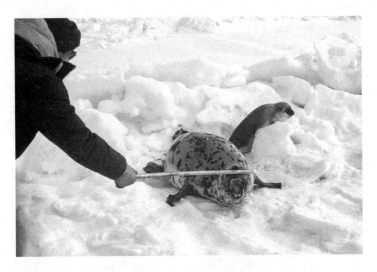

Wayne King checks a seal before getting too close.

25 minutes when feeding, we never kept them under anywhere near that time but injected the antidote as soon as possible. All recovered easily.

Tagging the males was a slightly different story. The dominant bulls generally stayed close to the females, which came into heat shortly after pupping. We had been watching one big fellow and eventually darted him. He was clearly the dominant male in the area and had chased others away. As the others approached, he threatened them with head high and hood bobbing, often with the red sac inflated. But the drugs made him too sleepy to display, and the pretenders to the throne received no threat as they approached. So we had to protect our client and his turf from another male that twice made forays to usurp "The Boss," who was clearly off his game. Hooded seals are not easily intimidated, even by vertical intruders, but we got him to retreat into the water both times. "The Boss" showed no gratitude when he recovered.

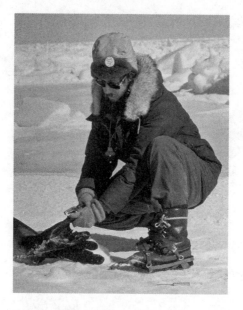

Rob Stewart applies a tag.

Our scariest moment came when a big male that must have received an inadequate dose headed for a lead, which is a narrow opening in the ice. We chased him, and Rob and Pierre-Yves took the brave step of grabbing his hind flippers while I injected antidote into the huge vein near his rear. Luckily he did not turn to attack, and the antidote began to work within 20 seconds. If he had made it into the water without the antidote, he may not have survived, although that is only speculation. As we let him go, he slid into the water seemingly none the worse for wear.

We made sure to keep the helicopter in sight at all times. The idea of becoming lost out there among the jagged ice mounds was not appealing.

Our helicopter pilot (I'll call him Fred) was quite a character, both feisty and a ladies' man. One morning we learned that he had been involved in a confrontation,

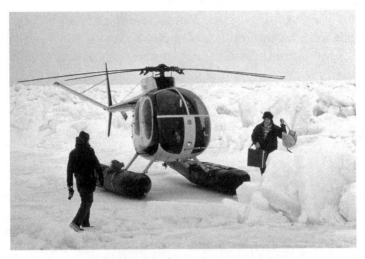

Helicopter among the ice mounds

nearly a fistfight, with some sealers who thought we were animal rights activists there to harass them. He was only about 165 centimetres (5 feet 4 inches) tall, but had the temperament of a terrier. On the Friday evening before we left the area, we all headed to a local pub for some R&R.

Near the end of our enjoyable evening, Fred disappeared with an attractive and lively young teacher whom we had met as we stood around the piano. The evening was memorable because of the warm and friendly atmosphere, the good beer and the wonderful mix of Acadian, English and French music. Much of it was fiddle tunes, but there had also been some sing-along songs that we all knew. The girl, who came from Nova Scotia, had been teaching in a school at one end of the island chain. Friday night was her night out, and she was desperate for some company. She explained that in her little community everybody not only knew everybody but also was related to everybody, which created some interesting teaching challenges. She and Fred hit it off at once. I guess a good-looking helicopter pilot wins hands down in the sex-appeal stakes.

Our return trip to the mainland was a great deal simpler than the outward journey. Fred ferried us across to Charlottetown in the evening, and the next morning we boarded Air Canada flights for home.

Both Rob and Pierre-Yves have gone on to spectacular and rewarding careers with marine animals, and seals have been a good part of that life. Rob, now retired, worked all over the Arctic in his time with the Department of Fisheries and Oceans. Pierre-Yves is a wildlife vet and member of the faculty at the Atlantic Veterinary College in Charlottetown. He is also the local coordinator for the important cross-country Canadian Wildlife Health Cooperative.

As he said to me when we reminisced about our trip, "What goes around comes around. Work on seals has now become a major part of my professional life!"

A Battering Encounter

Not all the urgent calls came in from folks near the city. Dr. Art Schatz, a colleague from the town of Wainwright, Alberta, three hours west of Saskatoon, called to ask for help with an unusual case—unusual to both of us.

A client of his had purchased two muskoxen because he had seen some them in the wild during a trip to the Arctic and was fascinated. Art told me that his client was worried about the female because she had a lame foreleg and could hardly walk.

I knew nothing of the muskox. A quick look at the college library's copy of *Mammals of Canada* told me some facts. The muskox lives in Canada's Arctic. It has an impressive long, hairy coat, and the skull is massive, as are the horns of the male. I felt a small tickle of concern when I read the short phrase, "The bulls charge each other head on." From the illustration and the information about the horns, I thought that might prove interesting. In Jasper we had seen footage of bighorn sheep

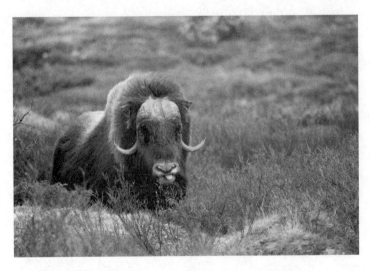

A muskox in natural habitat during the brief Arctic summer

135

rams going at each other with considerable violence during the breeding season, so much so that the clash of horns can be heard a mile away. Would the larger muskox display the same behaviour outside the breeding season?

While the book's picture was impressive, it held nothing to the real thing. The animal looked like a dark, overgrown version of the ultimate shaggy dog with a different head and a coat hanging almost to the ground. The horn boss of the bull was massive.

The darting went smoothly. But when Art and I reached the female, lying about 33 metres (108 feet) from the fence and three times that from the corral that held her consort, we heard some loud bangs as the bull expressed his displeasure at our actions. He was thumping one of the vertical 10- x 10-centimetre (4- x 4-inch) posts. We reckoned we did not have much time to examine and treat the animal. We were right. As I injected her with an antibiotic, we heard a loud crack, and the post buckled like a strand of wet spaghetti. As I administered the antidote to our patient, the bull broke through and galloped at us. Our hurdling technique over the fence might not have won any points for style, but style was irrelevant in this situation.

We retired to the truck. The furious bull ran right past the cow, continuing on to the fence. Having made his point, he snorted and turned back to stand beside his partner, just in case we might be foolish enough to make another sortie.

CHAPTER 14

A Bear Cub and a Dog

I could almost set my calendar every year in late March or early April to a call from the Provincial Department of Natural Resources (DNR) about orphaned black bear cubs found somewhere up north. The year 1980 was no exception, but the cubs arrived in early February, a lot sooner than usual.

Knowing that all North American bears have an unusual reproductive cycle was a clue. Black bears breed in midsummer but the embryo goes into a state of "suspended animation," more correctly known as delayed implantation. This tiny collection of cells, the blastocyst, floats freely in the womb, fuelled by the fluids inside until it "decides" (by a mechanism that has not yet been explained) to attach to the uterine wall. The implantation occurs at about the time the mother goes into her winter den, but will only occur if she is in good condition. If she is severely undernourished, the embryo will almost certainly be resorbed. If things go well, the embryo will become the tiny bundle of fur that is born a month or two later, most often in late January or early February.

At birth the cubs are tiny and almost unable to walk. The family stays in the den for some time, the cubs nursing as needed and gradually growing stronger until they are ready to go exploring with mum. They stay with her until they are about a year and a half old.

This mother bear cannot have understood what the terrible noise she could hear actually was. No doubt the growling diesel engine was a sound she knew but probably did not associate with danger. What she could not have known was that this particular diesel was a huge earthmover clearing an area around her den to prepare it for a mining camp. Suddenly she was crushed to death by tons of earth, rock and trees.

The driver of the enormous machine must have been right on the ball because he was quickly out of his cab to see what damage he had wrought. He found two tiny cubs nestled against the sow's chest, both alive and almost certainly mewling. He must have been horrified.

It was late January and bitterly cold, with daytime highs hovering around –20ºC (–4ºF) while at night it dipped below –30ºC (–22ºF). An adult bear spending much of her time in the den would develop a cozy fug—that warm, smoky, stuffy atmosphere so favoured by the British—so this temperature would be no challenge. She could easily keep her cubs warm and snuggled up as they lay between her front legs or on her chest where they could easily suckle nourishing milk from one of her two teats, which like a human's are level with the armpits.

The orphaned cubs, which would have looked so tiny and helpless against their mother's breast, weighed no more than 700 grams (1.5 pounds). Their eyes were still closed, and their umbilical cords hardly dry. They would have had no chance of living even a full day.

He acted right away, no doubt on the radio installed in his cab (no cell phones in 1980). With admirable speed, someone on the crew bundled the cubs up in a warm blanket and headed to Saskatoon, some 400 kilometres (250 miles) away.

I was out walking my morning rounds, clad in winter boots, insulated trousers, parka and warm mitts all topped with a hood and toque when the zoo truck rumbled up. Brent was driving and invited me to hop in, and he explained that two tiny cubs were at the barn and needed attention.

It was obvious we had a real challenge at hand. The smallest cub was moribund, hardly responding and making no noise. It died within a couple of hours. The eyes of the larger cub, a male, were closed and a 10-centimetre (4-inch) length of dried umbilical cord was attached to its belly. On the zoo scale, it weighed less than 1 kilogram (2.2 pounds), so the driver had been right on, even without benefit of a scale. Perhaps he was from the north and an experienced fisherman, which would have been no surprise given that Saskatchewan has over 100,000 lakes, most full of fish. If my reference books were correct, this meant that the cub might have doubled its birth weight and could have been as much as two weeks old, which would make him an early arrival indeed.

Bottle raising bear cubs was nothing new to us, and in the past year we had raised two after they arrived from logging camps where their mothers had been raiding and were shot because they attacked staff members. Those cubs were much further along on their development and weighed 2 or 3 kilograms (4.4 to 6.6 pounds) by the time they reached us.

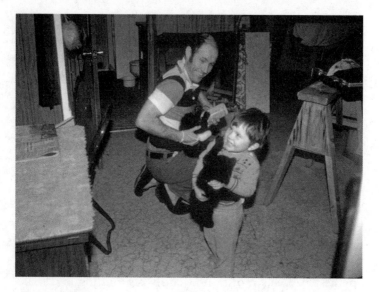

The weightlifter

My family helped out with the bottle raising, taking the two little cubs into our home. Of course the excited kids joined in, Karen having no trouble, but Charles was a tad too small to actually hold both bottle and bear.

Jo had returned to her medical career after two years of being a stay-at-home mum to raise our children, and work hours as a junior member of staff were pretty crazy. She was on duty every other night. But Celia, who had seen the bear explode the water container the previous summer, took to the task of feeding the cubs with enthusiasm. It is not every au pair girl from the English midlands who gets to feed bear cubs from a bottle every few hours!

We also had a new kitten we named Puss-in-Boots, and we restricted the pair to the basement, or rumpus room as it was called in those days. Rumpus it became once the kitten and the cubs got going.

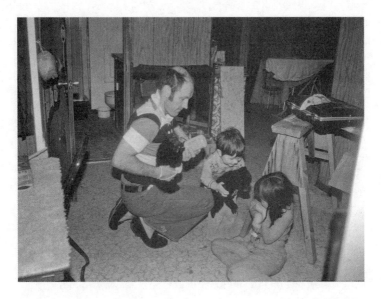

In the basement with Karen, Charles and our new tenants; in the late 1970s sideburns were "in."

The tiny newcomer orphaned by the earthmover accident was too small to take home and feed regularly. Another solution was needed.

Unfortunately, Celia had gone back to England, and with the kids in school we could not take this little guy home. Sharon, a full-time employee, diluted an evaporated milk product with some water and fed the bear in small amounts every three hours. After each feed she used a damp cloth to help him eliminate, and all seemed well at the beginning. The new cub showed a real tenacity and would most likely survive if nothing went wrong. It was soon obvious, however, in terms of being able to function and especially sleep, that the workload was a major challenge for Sharon and her colleagues. She more or less adopted the cub and even took it home for a weekend in

141

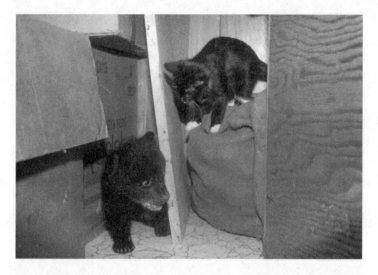

A new playmate for Puss-in-Boots, or is it the other way around?

order to keep up the feeding schedule. But she soon began to look distinctly jaded as a result of the crazy hours.

Then came a light-bulb moment. Could a foster-mother be found for this little guy to take the worst of the burden off our staff, particularly Sharon? I knew from something that Jo told me when we were first married that white elephant calves were revered, even worshipped, in some Asian and Indian cultures. Such calves were sometimes raised by a team of human wet nurses. My knowledge of the milk intake required by a 90-kilogram (200-pound) elephant calf, as opposed to a mere 3- or 4-kilogram (7- to 9-pound) human baby, caused my imagination to create a line-up of a gorgeous rainbow-coloured array of sari-clad mothers, like butterflies in a tropical garden doing a tag-team act.

One of the most remarkable examples of this particular form of cross fostering used to occur in Siam (now Thailand). In his 1931 book *Siamese State Ceremonies: Their History and Function: With Supplementary Notes*, Horace

Geoffrey Quaritch Wales documented the god-like position held by the king and described in great detail the reverence afforded to any white elephant and the rewards given to any person who found one and brought it to his majesty:

> …*I may add that it was formerly the custom to provide young White Elephants with a large number of human wet-nurses. I have in my possession a photograph, taken about a dozen years ago, of a Siamese woman suckling a young elephant, probably a white one.*

There are other similar accounts from Burma. Shelby Tucker, in the book *Among Insurgents: Walking Through Burma*, recorded the reverence afforded white elephants and stated that the Burmese ladies competed for the privilege wet-nursing these animals.

Other human–animal wet nurse stories come to mind. The classic, which may be more myth than fact, is the story of the founders of Rome, brothers Romulus and Remus, who were nursed by a she-wolf. There are plenty of other records of humans nursing animals. For example, as reported by Samuel Radbill in 1976: "travellers in Guyana observed native women breastfeeding a variety of animals, including monkeys, opossums, pacas, agoutis, peccaries and deer."

When it comes to bears, I later learned that women are known to have wet-nursed abandoned polar bear cubs. I had read about this before, and so a return to Samuel Hearne's *A Journey to the Northern Ocean* was in order. His account of his times as an agent of the Hudson's Bay Company between 1768 and 1773 was the key. He not only reported about the domestication of many moose near Churchill, but wrote about the suckling of polar bear cubs:

*It is common for the Southern Indians to tame and domesti-
cate the young cubs; and they are frequently taken so young that
they cannot eat. On those occasions the Indians oblige their
wives who have milk in their breasts to suckle them. And one of
the company's servants, whose name is Isaac Batt, willing to be
as great a brute as his Indian companions, absolutely forced one
his wives, who had recently lost her infant, to suckle a young
Bear.*

Other references come from reports about women of
the Ainu people of far northern Japan and the Itelmens
of Russia's Kamchatka Peninsula. How they managed the
sharp little teeth is beyond my imagination.

We knew that feeding the little cub every three hours,
day and night, was impossible. It became a case of trying
to find a suitable lactating female (not a human) to be the
milk donor. In those pre-laptop, pre-Google days of 1980,
but having some knowledge of this practice, I said to
Brent, "let me call Dr. Olfert at the animal resource centre
at the university to see if we can get some help."

We were in luck. Dr. Olfert said that a terrier-cross
female had just whelped and that we could borrow her for
the unusual task of raising our little orphan.

The zoo van was quickly on its way to the campus, and
an hour later the little family was safely settled in the barn,
with plenty of straw bedding. I was unsure if the dog
would accept the newcomer to her cute litter of four
mainly white pups, with the only black on them being
around their heads and ears. Although I have later learned
that dogs will often accept such newcomers without the
aid of drugs, it seemed prudent to sedate her and try to
fool her into thinking that nothing unusual had happened
when she awoke.

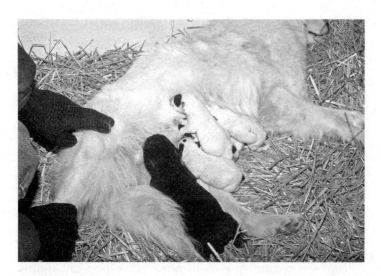

The milk bar is open.

The injection soon had her dozing soundly. Next I smeared over the little cub a bit of the feces that I had collected at his foster mum's rear end. He took no notice. The objective was to try and fool her into thinking he was one of hers and needed a cleanup. When the hungry cub was placed at her belly he at once latched onto a teat and began to suck as if there was no tomorrow.

Even before she was fully awake, she began to check on her litter. She licked both cub and pups. He was just one of the gang. He soon perked up, and within a week was having a good time, mixing with the pups, rolling, play-growling and so on, although in a slightly different language than his "litter-mates."

All went well for about four weeks, until on my daily check-ups it became obvious that the new mother's udder looked sore. On closer examination it appeared that her foster child's needle-sharp claws might be causing the problem. She seemed to be uncomfortable as soon as he began to feed, and we needed to do something before she rejected him outright.

It is unlikely that a five-week-old bear cub has ever had its toenails clipped, but that is what we did. While Sharon held the squirming little guy, I used a set of human nail clippers to do the job. His nails, sharp as needles, were quite short so care was the order of the day. A cut too far back would damage the nail bed. Other than the cub struggling and squawking a bit, the process went smoothly, unlike some dog clipping wrestling matches I engaged in during my general practice days in Kenya. We also wrapped the ends of his feet in sticky tape to try to further protect the female's udder and put him back with his buddies.

This worked for only two more days, then she simply turned off the taps. One day the pups and the cub were nursing, the next she would have nothing to do with them. It's probable that the cub's tiny needle-sharp teeth may have finally led to their dismissal, but the pretty little dog's job was done. She went home with all but one of her charges to Dr. Olfert's care at the university.

We weighed the cub every three days, and he had made great progress, stretching the spring to over 2 kilograms (4.4 pounds). He would need more milk for a while, and so we went back to the standard evaporated milk for bear cubs, but only three times a day, which was feasible for Sharon and her colleagues.

He did lose weight for three days, but then the scale began to stretch every day, and within a month he was up to 5 kilograms (10.5 pounds).

We hung on to the pup for about another month as he and the cub had formed a bond and seemed to spend their days roughhousing, eating or sleeping curled up together. Within a couple of weeks, they lost interest in the milk

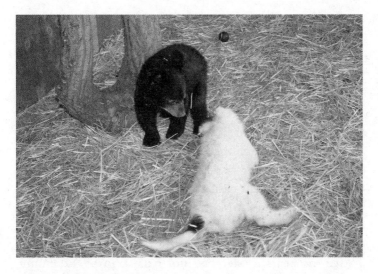

Playtime for pup and cub

because they found a much more enticing diet in the bowl full of milk, fruit and ground meat on offer.

The two buddies stayed indoors for another six weeks, the cub leaving the pup in the dust both literally when they played and weight-wise. On April 15, two and half months after he arrived, the bear cub weighed 15 kilos (33 pounds), almost as much as his foster mother when she adopted him.

By mid-April the weather warmed up, and two more cubs were in the outside run (with a good shelter attached). They had arrived from a logging camp where their unfortunate mother, like others before, had taken to terrorizing the staff as she raided the kitchen area in early March. This was a much more "normal" time for these new arrivals and so the now not-so-little guy joined them. It took him only five days to become the alpha bear. He was first to the food bowl, and as he weighed a bit more than his pen mates, he bossed them around without hesitation if he thought they had overstepped his rules.

There is a sad ending to this and other bear events at the Forestry Farm zoo during the time I served as the veterinarian there.

Each year, as soon as the children went back to school in early September, the now half-gown cubs were disposed of. Many went to a hunt ranch in the U.S., but when that operation no longer wanted them, they were simply shot. My protests fell on deaf ears. The most unfortunate of these shootings occurred the day before the Zoo Society's Lesley Avant came to the zoo with a group of young children. One of the highlights of the visit was to be a chance to see the bears. Lesley had not been told of the culling decision.

Perhaps I was being unrealistic. First of all, the pen was quite unsuitable for anything larger than a six-month-old bear. Second, they had been brought in on compassionate grounds, and to excite the children. And when the small visitors went away, the zoo could not continue to house the bears.

Even today zoos struggle with the successes of their breeding programs. A worldwide Facebook campaign about the culling of a giraffe at the Copenhagen zoo that garnered 30,000 signatures within a few days highlighted the problem of surplus animals. What does a zoo with creatures that can no longer be sheltered, either for economic reasons or because they can no longer contribute to the genetic pool that so many responsible zoo managers work with?

Keeping a giraffe in captivity is an expensive business with many dollars a day required on food supplies alone. On top are keeper's wages, barn heating, veterinary work and so on.

In a Times.com online article of February 10, 2014, titled *Marius The Giraffe Is Not The Only Animal Zoos Have Culled Recently*, Lisa Abend opens with this statement: "The killings of animals including zebras and pygmy hippos are necessary for conservation, zookeepers say, leading to mandatory euthanization in an effort to ensure there's room for other species, especially ones that need special protection."

The article is accompanied by the remarkable picture of a big male lion tearing at the carcass of a reticulated giraffe. Abend adds more species to her list, and these come from European zoos. They include "zebra, antelopes, bison, pygmy hippos, and tiny Red River hog piglets." Leopard cubs and other pig species are also listed.

At the Forestry Farm, in these more enlightened times, the only bears in the collection are a pair of orphaned and fully human-habituated grizzlies, and they live in a new enclosure that provides as much space as is feasible. They would probably have no clue how to survive in the wild and would also be a hazard if released because they would terrify and possibly attack anyone who might have the misfortune to encounter them.

CHAPTER 15

Bison Farming

The commercial production of bison in the meat and hide industry (as opposed to tourism) ranges from small units bordering on the hobby farm to huge operations. Farms with the least number usually have less than 10 head. At this scale, these folks cannot hope to make more than a small proportion of their annual income. Others who run between 20 or 30 head may make a decent return on investment when prices for stock are high and feed costs are down. Serious bison farmers and ranchers may have hundreds of breeding cows. If the percentage of these females that calve each year is high (upwards of 90) and sales are good, some owners can make a respectable income.

My first encounter with farmed bison occurred six weeks after my arrival in Saskatoon. A blond young enthusiast arrived and asked to speak to the "new bison guy" as Marie in reception announced over the phone. He proceeded to

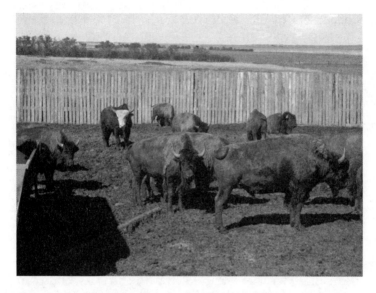

Bison/beefalo feedlot with a single beefalo with the white face of a Hereford

harangue me about the values of the crossbred beefalo (a cross between bison and cattle) that he was raising. He even took me to his farm for a tour.

It was clear that he was trying to convince me of their value and wanted a professional endorsement. I never heard from him again, but it wasn't long before I was visiting a bison farm to deal with a sick animal.

The first impression of the shambolic yard told a great deal. Several old sheds covered in the remains of what had once been a coat of red paint leaned over drunkenly. A pile of tangled barbed wire and used lumber studded with bent nails sat near the rusted carcass of an old tractor that looked as if it had been cannibalized for spare parts. Grass and weeds stuck up their heads among the mess. A man dressed in heavily worn and patched bibbed coveralls stepped out of the small wooden home. He asked me to take look at one of his nine cows; she was "off-colour."

The farmer ran the sorry-looking cow into a cattle squeeze. She offered no resistance, which was quite different from the behaviour of our zoo bison. After a clinical examination, I still could not figure out a specific reason for her condition, but something was obviously wrong. I took the shotgun approach of injecting an antibiotic, but I was not optimistic of the outcome.

A look at the blood sample in the lab at the college told me that she had a severe infection, so it was no surprise, three days later, to hear from the farmer that he was bringing the carcass to the college for a post mortem. Even today, 40 years later, I marvel that the bison lived as long as she did. Her liver was riddled with abscesses, and right in the midst of them was a piece of wire 15 centimetres (6 inches) long.

A different situation occurred about 70 kilometres (43 miles) north of the city. During several visits over the course of two years, a client (I'll call him Jonathan) called about minor problems. Jonathan had built a makeshift handling chute that threatened to fall apart every time an animal entered. It did allow him to get his females in for a pregnancy check, but a bull could have turned the chute into kindling in short order. With only 12 head, bison farming was more of a hobby for Jonathan. His main source of income was the car dealership he owned in the nearby town.

Jonathan seemed to be living a dream of his granddad's life as a pioneering homesteader. From a seat on rustic furniture inside his attractive bungalow, I admired the old one-point, horse-drawn plough sitting on the floor and the somewhat rusted scythe mounted above the fireplace. The view through the picture window showed gorgeous yellows, reds and greens of fall leaves reflected as blurry lines in the North Saskatchewan River.

Jonathan had built the robust bison-proof fence in such a way that it was not visible from the house, but rather along a shallow dip in the ground. The fence was fine but it enclosed only three sides of the field.

He called one day with desperation evident in his voice, to tell me that the neighbour wanted the bull removed from his herd of purebred Hereford cattle. It had routed the prize bull and was paying far too much attention to the cows. When I got to the farm, I realized how the escape had happened. The bull, no doubt drawn by irresistible scents wafting downwind, had simply swum across the river, jumped or crashed through a three-strand barbed wire fence and taken over the harem. Jonathan had obviously forgotten that bison of yore likely crossed innumerable rivers during their migrations over the centuries.

He had a horse trailer hitched to a half-ton in the yard to bring back the fugitive. I piled into his truck, and we crossed the road bridge 10 kilometres (4 miles) downstream and then headed back south along the grid road to the neighbour's place, where he was waiting with a sturdy young man.

The cows took little notice of the truck and trailer. They must have seen one like it dozens of times. A few even approached us, thinking that we had some goodies, maybe oats, on board. Of course, other cows were not going to miss out, and the bison bull followed the entire herd. He was not going to give up his hard won prizes that easily. The dart hit him in exactly the right spot, and five minutes later he was down and out. Then came the problem: How were four of us going to get 800 kilograms (1760 pounds) of immobile bison into the back of a horse trailer?

We grunted and groaned. The ramp helped a bit, but we eventually had to run a stout rope through the front of the trailer, loop it around the bull's chest and use the truck as a winch. That made life a lot easier, although I was worried about the bull's position on his side. As soon as he was past the tailgate so that we could close, it I gave him an anti-dote and waited nervously to see and hear what came next. It was not long before we heard thrashing sounds and saw the metal sides of the trailer move in and out in response to his efforts to stand or his objection to confinement. Afterwards it was a case of taking the reverse route across the bridge and back to the "homestead."

Another trip to a bison farm took place in Hawaii, a popular holiday destination for many folks from Saskatchewan, especially in winter. My trip was neither for a holiday, nor in winter. It was late October and the annual conference of The American Association of Zoo Veterinarians made a visit to that state and was exactly what I needed. We shared and learned new things. We met old friends and made new ones. In the evenings we sat on the beach, enjoyed a beer or two and watched the glorious sunsets. We also visited the zoo.

I also got the chance to do something a bit different. I had been corresponding with Bill Mowry, who had a bison operation on the north side of the island of Kauai. He wanted my support in his endeavours to import breeding stock and was running into some bureaucratic roadblocks. When I told him of our upcoming gathering, he invited some of my colleagues and me to visit his Hanalei ranch. Of course we went, five of us sharing the cost of chartering a small plane.

Bill picked us up and took us to his home for the first order of business, lunch. Bill's wife, Marty, had laid on a meal as we sat on the veranda of their bungalow and admired the view of the ocean. As we enjoyed the avocado with vinaigrette, a sudden downpour rattled the roof.

Bill explained, "We get over 80 inches [200 centimetres] per year. This is the wettest place on earth."

After the meal, we joined him in a walk to see the bison. The first thing that struck me were the three lush paddocks, each one pie-shaped with the sharp ends meeting at a single set of handling yards.

We learned that the grass and alfalfa mix stayed green all year. Bill simply rotated the animals through the yards and out to new grazing pastures with a simple technique.

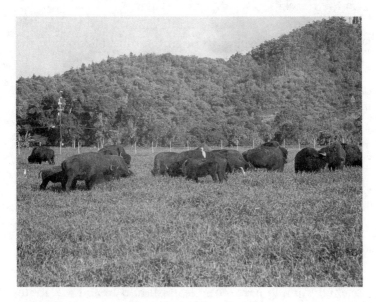

Bison knee deep in lush pasture

He closed the gate to the field they were in for a couple of days. That kept them out of the corral that housed the only source of water. After two days, they all lined up to get in. He then opened the gate to the next paddock in the rotation and let the herd into the corral. He showed us how it was a simple matter to pull a cable and close the gate they had just come through.

My Australian friend and colleague, Tony English, asked about parasites, imagining that the crowded and moist conditions would be a paradise for worms. Bill had an elegant solution. There was a sheltered walkway above one gate, which was only 2.5 metres (8 feet) wide. The walkway had a rainproof roof and a slatted floor. The animals had to pass under the slatted floor to get to the narrow gate, which they could get through only two by two. Bill sat on the slatted floor and simply poured the dewormer on their backs as they passed through.

The relentless year-round rainfall meant that by the time he had moved the herd through the third paddock in the circle the first one had new growth ready to graze.

As for the permit, I heard no more.

~

Even farther afield and much less likely was a trip to Australia to visit a bison farm. The country proved surprising for a naïve Canadian who had read about its geography, watched its cricketers and seen pictures of kangaroos, wombats and a host of other creatures unique to the continent. I was invited to speak at a deer conference in the town of Albury, in the state of New South Wales. As we sat over an evening beer, Tony English told Jo and me about his work with other species.

"You know we have a bison farm near here, don't you," he said.

This was news. One phone call and two mornings later, we headed east from Albury. After an hour and a half's drive through rolling hills, we reached the farm owned by Ashley and Deanne Brown. Dave Hall, the local vet, arrived, and we chatted about the problems of getting the animals into the country.

Ten years before our visit, Ashley had sourced his start-up herd from three different ranches in Canada. Later, he acquired a bull from the U.S. Given the tough restrictions on livestock imports that the Australians need to impose to prevent any new diseases arriving, there must have been some interesting bureaucratic exchanges.

Ashley told us that one of the cows needed treatment. She had tangled her hind leg in the fence, and Dave had to amputate the foot. Ashley's task was to catch the animal so that Dr. Hall could change the bandage and give an anti-biotic injection. I was interested to see how much the handling system that Ashley used resembled the ones in North America. I assumed our task would be to help herd the bison into corrals so that the patient could be dealt with in a chute. I was wrong. Ashley emerged from the house carrying a longbow and an arrow with a dart at the business end. I had read about these bow and arrow darting systems but had never seen one.

We walked out into a paddock where the bison cows were contentedly grazing. The scene might have been anywhere, with two exceptions. We were in the southern hemisphere, so the snow and brown grass of late fall at home were absent. Here the animals were grazing on spring green. The other exception was the tree species. Tall gums formed the backdrop.

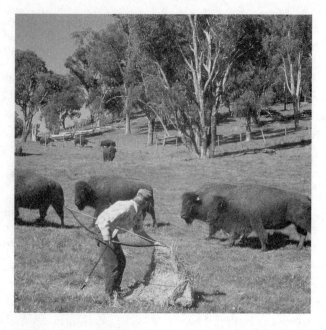

Ashley's bow-and-arrow darting system; gum trees in the background

Ashley calmly walked out into the middle of the field and waited beside the remains of a hay bale that had been used for winter-feeding. The animals walked past without a care in the world. Most of them took no notice of the archer.

With the drugs duly delivered the rest of the process went smoothly.

CHAPTER 16

From Farm to Ranch

For students in their final year, the college offered two- or four-weeklong rotations in several veterinary-related disciplines. By 1999 I was no longer doing any zoo work, so the former zoo rotation was replaced by two others—game ranching and free-ranging wildlife.

The wildlife rotation comprised one-month externships in Uganda. The game ranching rotation was more local, but it covered only Saskatchewan and Alberta. Students could sign up to visit and work at farms where "alternative livestock" were managed for commercial purposes. On each rotation they would see and treat at least two species of deer (elk, white-tailed, reindeer or fallow) and at least two bison farms.

The oddest examples of all these alternative farms were those raising ostrich and emu. At that time, the ostrich industry was at its peak. Prices for a breeding pair reached as high as $80,000. The return on investment was the large number of eggs sold at high prices to new famers hoping to cash in.

There were, and still are, many bison farms in both provinces. The best-designed and managed farm among the many I visited and worked at over the years belonged to John and Ginny Grinde, which was six hours west of Saskatoon near Rimbey, Alberta.

The chance to visit the farm and take a few students every year came about because John contacted me. His first request had nothing to do with bison but was about John wanting to keep up his veterinary licence in his home province. He had graduated from the Western College of Veterinary Medicine in Saskatoon in 1974, the year before I arrived. He called out of the blue to ask if he could spend some time with me to gain some new experiences. This "mentoring" under the supervision of a veterinarian is required in most countries to make sure professional standards are maintained.

We planned John's visit for one of the two weeks scheduled for the game ranching rotation so that he could work on deer and other species. During our time together, we had many discussions beyond those about the deer and bison operations. Inevitably the ostrich phenomenon was part of the conversation. We agreed that it was really a pyramid scheme in which early adopters could make small fortunes quickly. Over and above that was the little matter of climate. I told him about a case one winter, during the peak of the ostrich boom, when an unusual but not really surprising case arrived at the vet school. A cock ostrich had such severe frostbite that he had no sensation or living tissue for 30 centimetres (12 inches) up his legs. The result was inevitable, and I have no idea how much the client lost on his investment.

We also visited hobby farms where llamas were raised. None of the students knew much about them, so the information gleaned was useful because the students would probably encounter them or their cousins, the alpaca, in their careers. In time farmers realized that alpaca wool was far superior to that of llamas, and a changeover occurred. The odd thing about these two species is that the Incas of the high Andes Mountains domesticated them at least 4000 years ago, but in North America they are classed as an alternative species.

As we worked together, John realized the importance of teaching and exposing soon-to-be vets to new experiences. He also offered me the chance to take students to his ranch where he ran about 100 head of breeding cow bison and a feedlot of 500 to 700 head to supply the meat market. He suggested that the students would get an opportunity to be involved in hands-on work if we visited when he was doing his annual vaccinations and de-worming.

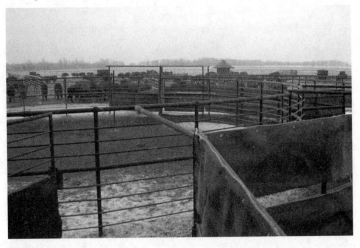

The circular sorting pen with an alley outside it and the holding pens outside

By September of the following year everything was in place. After the long drive, students and professor pulled up past a well-tended vegetable garden and stopped beside two vehicles, a red, flatbed half-ton truck and a grey Saturn sedan.

We had two days of intense work using John's elegantly designed, built and welded handling system, which was simple to operate. From the paddocks, he brought the animals into a series of pie-shaped pens. They were set like the arms of a clock around a circular sorting pen in the middle. Each arm had a stout gate that led to an alleyway into which the now-subdivided herd was persuaded to go. Three or four students carried out this part of the process.

Once the bison were in the alleyway it was easy to push them into the sorting pen with the farm tractor and a large board slightly narrower than the alley itself.

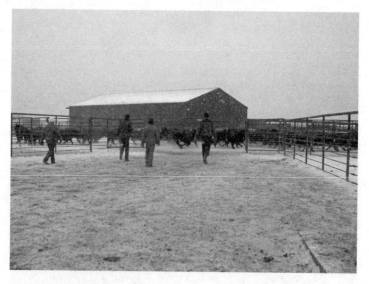

Students "persuading" the bison to enter the alleyway

John stood sorting for the first run to show everyone what to do. He closed the gate as some of the animals ran past. After the demonstration, a student did the job each time.

As the animals ran in a counter-clockwise direction, they went through the open shed door into a semi-circular series of in-line paired metal panels. The space between the panels was narrow enough to ensure that the bison stood one behind another. One of the team closed the sliding door behind the last animal to enter. The rest of the job was relatively easy.

At the other end of the line of panels stood the custom designed squeeze chute operated by a hydraulic system. At the back, as the animal entered, a door slid shut behind it. The walls could be adjusted so that each animal was held without being overly crushed.

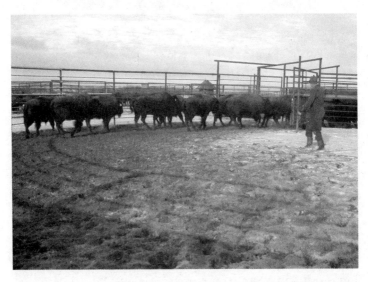

John cuts out a small number so that they can be brought into the shed.

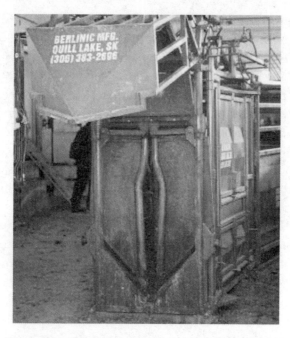

The squeeze chute ready to go. The crash gate is shown in the elevated position. It is lowered before an animal enters.

At the front a head gate stood partially open, making the bison think it might be able to go forward and return to its paddock. However, a crash gate situated in front of the head gate stopped the animal cold. Once a bison was in position, we had a series of procedures to follow. All the cows were checked for pregnancy, and every animal was vaccinated against blackleg, a potentially fatal condition, and treated with de-wormer.

Once the procedures were complete, the bison was released, jumping forward out of the squeeze and hightailing it out and away.

Sadly, John died of cancer in 2012. Part of his obituary reads: "family man, friend, farmer, veterinarian, paddler,

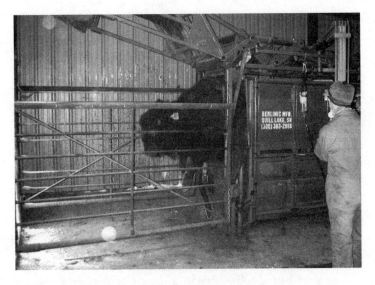

John lifts the crash gate, and off she goes.

outdoorsman, businessman." He was a very special man. He is greatly missed, not only by his family but by all who knew him.

Twelve years before he died, John and I attended the Bison 2000 conference in Edmonton where we heard the keynote speaker, billionaire Ted Turner, present his vision on the future of the industry. His involvement, as a ranch owner, lies at the peak of the commercial bison business. His power of speech and the message he gave were impressive. He predicted that the bison industry, which had already taken a downturn in the late 20th century, would continue to do so. Animals were being culled because the cost of production exceeded the returns.

One of the most fascinating moments of the conference was the after-dinner meeting when three First Nations chiefs sat with Mr. Turner on the raised stage. They presented him with a beautifully decorated bison hide. The four of them then shared a ceremonial pipe.

Mr. Turner's prediction turned out to be accurate. Prices did tank, but they have come back. As of 2015, bison meat has become more widely available in supermarkets and other outlets, as people have recognized the quality of the meat. This trend was heightened by Turner's foresight starting Ted's Montana Grill in the U.S., a restaurant chain with 49 locations featuring bison as one of the most sought-after menu items. Today, the supply from all sources cannot meet the increasing demand.

Mr. Turner, through Turner Enterprises is the owner of the largest number of bison, about 50,000 head held on 15 ranches across the U.S. He is also the owner of the second largest group of properties, approximately two million acres (809,371 hectares), in the U.S.

None of his ranches stocks animals at higher densities than the land will sustain. For example, the area of the Armendaris Ranch in the Chihuahuan Desert of New Mexico is 330,000 acres (133,546 hectares). The operation manages only 1000 head, meaning that bison can roam over several pastures. This low stocking rate does not damage the land. Many paddocks in less harsh landscapes are in the 10- to 12,000-acre (4500 hectare) range where the grazing and land type will sustain higher stocking rates. Each ranch develops a yearly grazing plan based on range assessments. Due to climate variations, stocking rates change based on estimated available forage in each paddock to prevent overgrazing or over utilization of the land. Many of the ranches are on a conservation easement that allows "sustainable and proper use" of the land.

Great care is taken to manage pasture. Some paddocks are left vacant for up to a year, allowing for full recovery of the pastures and parasite control. Most parasites are unable to survive a full calendar year without infecting an animal host, so when the bison returned to the unused paddock, they were able to graze on "clean" grass.

Wildlife veterinarian Dr. David Hunter is responsible for the health and welfare of the bison on Turner's ranches. His duties involve parasite control, vaccination protocols and the effects of management practices on reproductive rates. As he said to me, "There is no point in carrying cows that are barren. They simply consume the grazing and contribute nothing to the economic wellbeing of the business." And the operation has to be run as a business. The income from the ranching is vital for maintaining other aspects of Ted's vision.

Dr. Hunter is also involved in several conservation programs that range widely, including efforts to preserve Mexican gray wolves, prairie dogs, black-footed ferrets, Bolson tortoises, gopher tortoises and other species. The Turner Endangered Species Fund finances all of Hunter's work. The mission statement of Turner Ranches is "to manage Turner lands in an economically sustainable and ecologically sensitive manner while promoting the conservation of native species." His Endangered Species Fund website tells much of this story.

Turner is a bison rancher, but on all of his ranches he practices conservation. He cares about the land and the legacy of his efforts. He does his best to preserve the land and even return it to its natural condition. To achieve this goal, he must generate income, and a major part of that income comes from the bison operations.

Bison are a keystone species for land recovery. They provide food for top predators such as grizzly bears, black bears, mountain lions and wolves. The leftovers from these kills feed smaller predators such as coyotes, other smaller mammals and eventually carnivorous and scavenging birds as well as insects and bacteria.

Another aspect of the bison's keystone function is land use and food for herbivores. Bison keep the grass at sustainable heights, providing grazing for other species such as elk, mule deer, bighorn sheep and pronghorn antelope. Smaller animals also benefit. Prairie dogs can make their burrows, and these become homes to black-footed ferrets, burrowing owls and snakes. A vital part of the ecosystem is the fertilizing effect of dung and the provision of material for dung beetles to complete their life cycles.

According to statistics gathered by the Canadian Bison Association, more than 125,000 commercially raised plains bison are being grown on 1211 properties in the country. In addition, the Committee on the Status of Endangered Wildlife in Canada (COSEWIC) states that, as of 2013, five isolated, wild subpopulations of approximately 1200 to 1500 mature individuals roam across the land. More than 800 bison reside in zoos worldwide: 70 wood bison, 110 plains bison and the majority unclassified. No wood bison are held on farms or ranches. Currently, COSEWIC has calculated the population of wild wood bison at between 5000 and 7000 individuals, the majority living in the Mackenzie Bison Sanctuary in the Northwest Territories. It was in this population that a massive die-off occurred in 2012, the result of an anthrax outbreak.

According to the website of the National Bison Association in the U.S., approximately half a million plains bison roam in the country. Of these 16,000 live on public lands such as state parks. Yellowstone National Park has some 5000 head of the only truly free-ranging plains bison in the U.S.

∾

CHAPTER 17

Tarzan and Family

I n the popularity sweepstakes, Tarzan and his capuchin
monkey family tied with George and Queenie as the
most popular residents of our zoo. In summer, when
the sliding door to their pen gave them access to the outdoor south-facing, fully glassed-in section, visitors crowded
around to ogle for long periods as the monkeys sat around,
jumped from one bar to another or groomed themselves
and each other. School groups seemed to enjoy the sight
and ooh-ed and ah-ed and sometimes giggled as they
looked on.

In winter the three monkeys were confined indoors
except on relatively warm days when the sun was shining.
They are, after all, a tropical species native to Central and
South America. Many years later in Costa Rica, my wife
and I saw them roaming free and happy in Manuel Anto-
nio National Park. We were limited to the pathways, and

it felt as though *they* were watching us, not the other way around.

Tarzan was very much the alpha male. Not only was he twice as the size of the two females, his big, tough body, particularly his large round head with its heavy jaw muscles, made it clear he was the boss. It was his mounting of the females that caused the most reaction from the schoolchildren, and I was amused at the interesting ways their teachers dealt with explaining basic biology 101, or "doin' what comes naturally" as Irving Berlin wrote for his hit musical *Annie Get Your Gun*.

These monkeys had also come across from the Golden Gate, and although their new quarters were less than ideal they were surely better off than in their former home. John and Jureen, the two keepers who worked with the monkeys at the Golden Gate, made a real effort to enhance their environment by erecting rope swings, perches and

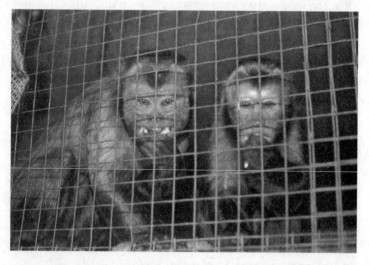

Chow time. Tarzan, at left, is about twice the size of his female companion.

a couple of baffles to give the little monkeys a chance to get out of line-of-sight of people or one another if they so wished.

There were no vaccines to administer that I knew of, and a routine check for fecal parasites came up negative likely because their omnivorous diet consisted of a variety of fruit and commercial monkey chow, none of which were likely to carry parasites. In the wild when the meat part of the diet includes insects, birds' eggs and even small vertebrates, some of these can act as intermediate hosts for disease agents.

Nobody knew if these monkeys were raised in captivity, but it seemed likely, as they did not exhibit any of the typical behaviours often seen in captive animals.

One thing was almost certain; the monkeys had never been tested for tuberculosis, a disease seen in several species of monkey, as well the great apes. Sadly, it is a disease of captive primates, rather than wild ones, and is well known in zoo collections. The risk to human keepers who come into regular contact with their charges is high.

None of the three showed any signs of disease, but it would not have been wise to ignore the need for testing. The process is quite simple, requiring a steady hand, an immobilized monkey, a super fine needle and an altered extract of the live tuberculosis bacterium that doesn't cause disease. The test protocol involves an injection of a tiny amount of the extract, called tuberculin, into the skin. In people, this is called the Mantoux test, and the injection is given on the inner aspect of the lower arm. In monkeys, the tuberculin is injected into of one of the eyelids of the patient, not through the thin skin but *into* it.

Having obtained one vial of tuberculin from the government veterinary office, I prepared to do the injections. With the blowgun now part of the basic zoo equipment it was not difficult to administer the anesthetic, but the challenge was that we had to do all three of the little guys in one session. None of them had ever seen a blowgun in action, so not even the smallest female was spooked with the puffing.

First we did a general physical and found nothing out of the ordinary. The skin of the eyelid is very thin, and it would have been easy to go through it, rendering the test useless. I used a 28-gauge needle, which is only a tad thicker than a human hair, to inject a single tiny drop of precisely one-tenth of one cc into each monkey's left lid.

Keepers John and Jureen had worked with the monkeys in their days at the Golden Gate and had no trouble differentiating between the two females. Not so for me or the rest of the crew. The solution was simple—use a small tattoo pen to make a small black dot above the eye on each animal, one on the right, the other the left.

Then we waited, checking the monkeys every day. On day two, the "left-dotted" female had a small swelling in the lid. On day three, her eye was almost shut, and the skin was redder than on the "normal" side.

The government vet came out later that morning to take a look. We both knew that other forms of tuberculosis could cause the same reaction. The most common, especially in captive primates, is called avian TB, which affects birds. We waited a month to let things settle, and at that point, the black dots came into play. We knew which of the two females needed the re-test but with a different protocol.

After she was once again anesthetized and bare patches were shaved on her chest, the government vet took over. He injected the same tuberculin on the left and the avian one on the right. On day three, all the keepers, Brent the foreman and even the park supervisor had taken a look at the monkey before I arrived. It was clear that the main reaction was limited to the right-hand side. Of course, the government vet needed to see the result. Had the red reaction been on the side linked to human TB, we would have a mass of paperwork to complete. In addition, every member of staff, even the gardening crew, would have to go through the test procedure. All would have been on tenterhooks worrying about our own TB status. The worry would have extended to our families, our occasional contacts, and maybe even theirs. We were all relieved.

Eighteen months later, Jureen announced that we had a new group member. The unnamed female with the dot above her right eye had given birth. Tarzan had rung the bell. Naturally we were all delighted. Soon after the happy event Jureen asked me to take a look at the two-week-old infant. He thought something was wrong with its tail. Fortunately, Jureen had been feeding the monkeys a few grapes every day and had gained their complete trust.

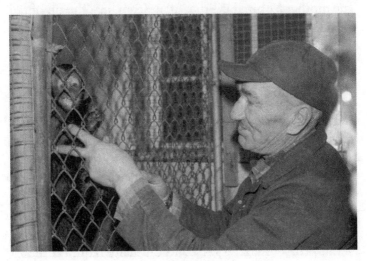

Jureen says hello.

When they saw him coming into the barn in the morning they would go right up to him, gripping the page wire of the pen and squeaking with what sounded like anticipation. If human kids are anything to go by, it might have been a demand. Perhaps it was a mixture of the two.

By this time, the adult monkeys seemed to have forgotten the insults heaped upon them during the repeated tuberculin testing. The mother stood next to Jureen, who had a handful of grapes ready. She came right up to the wire, the infant firmly attached to her belly. Jureen fed her the fruit, one piece at a time. I was able to see that the tip of its tail was dark, almost black and had no hair on it. It did not look good.

I told Jureen that we would watch them closely, checking every day. Two days later, grapes in my own hand, I took a closer look. The hairless end of the tail had now extended even farther towards the baby's backside.

Jureen, to my amazement, opened the door of the pen. The mother let him take the infant from her. The tip of tail was cold and swollen; it was gangrenous. I needed to act promptly.

We couldn't be certain how the infant had been injured, but Jureen thought that it might have been attacked by one of its pen mates. We had no way of knowing which of the three possible was the culprit—the mother, the other adult female or Tarzan. The easiest to eliminate was its mother. Tarzan was only a remote possibility; after all, the infant carried his DNA. That left the other female. She seemed to be a reasonable candidate, but we couldn't be sure. Jureen tucked the tiny infant inside his jacket, and we headed over to the clinic.

The protocol at the vet college usually required me to pass surgical cases on to the surgeons, but nobody was free for several hours, so I had to get on with the treatment myself. The patient had to get back to his mother as soon as possible. It would not be a complicated procedure; I'd done similar in my private practice days.

The surgery to remove the gangrenous end of the tail was simple. An injection of a small amount of local anesthetic about 4 centimetres (1.6 inches) above the junction eliminated any possibility of pain for the little guy. It was easy to judge where to cut because the live tissue was warm, the dead tissue cold. While we waited for the anesthetic to take effect, I filled a hot water bottle and placed it, wrapped in a towel, under the patient and another towel over top. Next, a rubber band, twisted a few times and slipped high up onto its tail made a handy tourniquet.

The key was to lop off enough tail at a junction between the tiny bones to ensure that everything left behind was healthy and had a blood supply. A flap of healthy skin on both sides was needed to fold over the stump for the stitches. All this took only a few minutes except for burying the sutures. Just like Jonjon in Kenya. If the monkeys, especially the mother, found any tag ends of nylon, they would promptly pull them out. Three stitches did the trick, and when all was done, we used a swab to wipe off the iodine and alcohol that had been used to prepare the surgical site.

Jureen stood quietly by as I explained what I was doing. Then with the monkey again tucked inside his jacket, we headed back to the barn. Jureen put the little guy back on a shelf in the cage. His mum came over, sniffed once and took off, heading to the far corner of the cage. This was not good. Had she detected the smell of the disinfectant, or perhaps of me?

Our next step was to let the other two back from the outer section of the display and leave them to themselves. We thought their presence might induce the mother to pick up her youngster as a protective or jealous act. Half an hour later, Jureen checked in. The infant had not moved and was cold to the touch. A rescue action was needed.

A syringe of my favourite cocktail and the blowgun did the trick on the mother, and she was soon asleep. We found a wooden box big enough to hold the pair of them and soon had a blanket in it. A 25-watt light bulb affixed to the wire front of the box made an ideal heater.

The next task was to eliminate what remained of the disinfectant smells. Washing with warm water was a start but it would probably not be enough. I dipped a Q-tip into the mother's mouth, another one into her rectum and smeared the result over the baby, including the upper end of its tail. Jureen placed the hungry infant against its mother's breast where it at once began to suckle, albeit rather weakly. An hour later we returned to check their progress. The mother was awake, and the baby was nestled against her. All was well. We breathed a sigh of relief for another successful outcome.

An Escape with a Bad Ending

During a summer night in 1980 someone with mischief in mind broke into the zoo grounds and jimmied the lock on the wolf pen. By the time any of us working with the animals arrived in the morning, police had shot all seven wolves. Their bloodied carcasses lay about the grounds like discarded rubbish. The park director had called the cops, and that was that. All of us who worked with the animals were angry and horrified. The anger stemmed from the fact that the director had not even called me. Such an action should have been a no-brainer. For the keepers, the anger was multiplied when the director accused them of leaving the gate open. He had not bothered to come out and take a look; he had just assumed without benefit of evidence.

Our horror was again intensified by the fact that I had been treating one of the pack, a human-raised orphan, with eye drops three times daily for four days for an eye infection. He would come to a call, just like a pet dog. If the director had bothered to read the daily reports, he would have known this.

CHAPTER 18

Pond Inlet
Part 1: Arrival

"There she is!" John called over the helicopter intercom. We were 2 kilometres (1.2 miles) east of the community of Pond Inlet (now Qikiqtaaluk) on the extreme North Eastern shore of Canada's Baffin Island. I was there at the invitation of Ray Schweinsburg, polar bear biologist for the Northwest Territories. Ray was one of several scientists around the world studying polar bear ecology. John Lee, his face partly concealed by a dark beard, was a wildlife technician and the second member of the team.

Our research work, which involved tagging bears for identification, began with good luck on the very first day. I looked down from my seat behind the pilot to see the small figure of a polar bear heading across the sea ice about 300 metres (985 feet) out from the cliffs to our right. Two tiny cubs followed behind her.

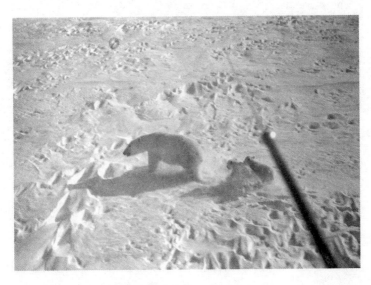

Cubs of the year with their mother

That first day, Ray stayed back in Pond Inlet to meet with Inuit elders about the program. John, pilot Tex Walker and I were at the start of a long day under ideal conditions. Ideal because, as John explained, "It snowed during the night, so any tracks we see will be fresh. A real opportunity will occur if we see a fresh seal carcass."

Next came two days of fatiguing, frustrating days on old snow when Ray, sitting up front beside Tex, tried to determine how old any set of prints might be and whether it was worth following them to see if we could find a bear.

The next day we tried to go out, but fog and snow made flying not just difficult, but outright dangerous. Tex called a halt not 20 minutes after take-off.

"I can't distinguish the difference between the ice surface and the cliffs," he said. "On top of that it's snowing, and I can't see the cliff tops either. It's too dangerous to fly and may get worse. We're heading back."

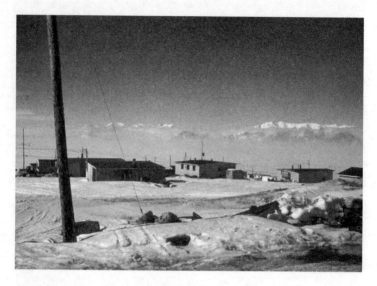

The village of Pond Inlet (Qikiqtualuk)

By noon the fog had lifted, giving me the chance to take a walk and refresh my memory of first impressions of the town and surrounding area. Many single story homes had snowmobiles and quad bikes parked beside them. Next to one home a caribou head with enormous antlers was evidence of successful hunt. Power poles rose all over the community. Several kamatiks, long wooden sleds lashed together with ropes, stood on the shore. A few kids rode by on their bicycles. The school, looking as if it was newly built, stood near the edge of town. With spring just around the corner, patches of dark rock, where the snow had melted, stood out. Away to the north, the cliffs of Bylot Island, the protected bird sanctuary, showed clearly.

That first day, however, even from 100 metres (330 feet), the tracks of the female and her cubs were obvious, so we dropped down to take a closer look. We could see, beside the dinner-plate sized indents in the snow, a mass of much

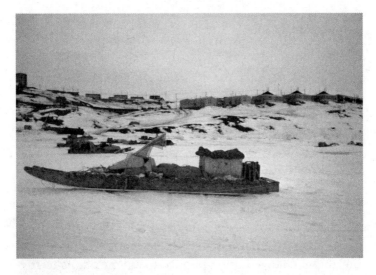

Kamatik

smaller prints. Within five minutes we closed in on the little family.

The call from Ray to take part in this polar bear project had come out of the blue. He had called, introduced himself and asked for my help with bear immobilization. They were looking for something to replace Sernylan in the work on polar bears with the Territorial Department of Wildlife.

Sernylan, which works very nicely on bears, had become a restricted drug because of street abuse (if you can imagine anyone stupid enough to take it). There are horrific stories about its abuse by people.

Ray had read about the work done in Canada's mountain parks and Prince Albert with a two-drug mixture of ketamine and a cattle sedative called Xylazine.

Faye Kernan, the college's pharmacist, was enthusiastic about the many new drug combinations needed for my wildlife work. She was up to the challenge and made up several new vials of the Ketamine/Xylazine concoction, which we shipped to Yellowknife. Before long, Ray and John reported success with the combination, noting that drugging big males was a problem because of the volume of the drug that needed to be injected. Some bears had to be injected twice.

At first the mixture worked well, and Ray and John published a scientific paper on the use of the drug combo, to which they added Faye's name and mine even though we did not directly participate in the sedation of the bears. But things changed. John phoned to tell me of one terrifying encounter:

We darted a young female with a maximum dose and followed her for a while. She didn't slow down, so we gave her a second dart. After a while more she did begin to drag her feet and then went down in about the normal five minutes or so that it takes for a dart to work. Ray and I both felt as if something was not quite right. We buzzed her, hovering right over her back for quite a while, but she didn't move. We even wondered if she was dead.

We landed about 40 metres [130 feet] or so away, and Tex shut the engine down to save fuel. In retrospect, that probably saved Ray from a bear wrestle/mauling, because the bear heard us approach before we got right on top of her. Ray climbed down from the left-hand door and walked round the bubble, bending under the radio antenna that stuck out like a swordfish bill, to my side. I also stepped down and we both followed safety protocols by having our firearms ready.

Ray had a pistol, a .44 magnum. I had a rifle. We chanted our usual mantra as we approached, "Hey bear, hey bear." When we were about 20 feet [6 metres] from her, the bear's head came around, and in a flash she was up and charging right at Ray.

Ray ran but looked back and tripped over a pressure ridge, filling his gun barrel and cylinders with snow in the fall, making it inoperable. The bear stopped about 6 feet [1.8 metres] away at this strange behaviour, and there they were nose-to-nose, eyeball-to-eyeball.

Routinely, as soon as we moved away from the chopper, I carried my gun cocked and at the "high ready" so I moved it the tiny extra bit to my shoulder and fired. Luckily the bear dropped, but only a couple of feet from Ray. She had been playing possum all along but fortunately didn't wait until we were closer to let us know that.

During my African experience, I had seen an occasional dart failure, usually because the emptying mechanism misfired, but two of them? That was an aberration.

John was so matter-of-fact about the event that it took a while for me to register how well he had reacted in an incredibly dangerous situation. At best, drugging darts take time to work, at least four or five minutes. The television portrayal of instantaneous collapse is just nonsense.

Lots of stories come out of Africa about encounters with lions, when men needed lightning reflexes, but I knew of none from the Arctic. Ray and his team got into many sticky situations and chancy encounters during their studies, but they always tried to err on the side of caution for the bear. Their goal was to save bears not kill them. No researcher likes being in a situation where he has to kill and only does so under dire circumstances, as in this case, when something that can go wrong, does.

After their terrifying encounter, which must have shaken both men to the core, it was understandable that John contacted me again to see what else they might try. I suggested an even more powerful version of fentanyl, the potent opioid drug that worked so well in Jasper and Prince Albert. Instead of being 100 times more potent than fentanyl, the figure for carfentanil is 10,000 times more potent. It also lasts longer. I had used it on a few moose, some wolves and two bears at the zoo.

The condition on the use of the drug was that I would accompany Ray and John because it was restricted to veterinary use. Since John had already asked me to join the team in the Arctic, that was a non-issue. As the work with free-ranging animals was what I loved most about my job, it was no hardship to agree, providing the Forestry Farm Park Zoo director had no problem with my brief absence.

So there I was, on my first trip to the far North, working on the ultimate northern carnivore, a major charismatic species outside Africa, vying with China's panda for the number-one spot in the hearts and minds of the public. Not to mention advertisers using the polar bear image in movie theatres and on television, including an inane ad for Coca Cola. Every time I see that ad, I wonder how many people know that polar bears and penguins occupy different poles—North and South respectively.

As we flew over the mother bear and her two cubs, I drew the drugs from their vials and saw Tex, our Vietnam vet chopper pilot, again pulling a cigarette from the left breast pocket of his coveralls and his Zippo lighter from the other. Once again, I worried as this seemed to be what he did every time we saw a bear and prepared to go into chase mode. The cigarette habit fitted precisely with his nicotine-stained fingers that ended in the most bitten-down nails I have ever seen. Perhaps his war experiences were memories best not thought about.

However nervous he may have felt inside, Tex took us quickly and cleanly alongside the mother bear, and I pulled the trigger. A fraction of a second later, a silver-coloured dart stuck out of her shoulder, and we were peeling away even as John growled, "Got her!" into the intercom.

Tex put the machine into a steady climb and circled downwind of the bears. Soon the mother bear slowed and then stopped. A minute later, she went down in a heap and lay stretched out on her side. The cubs moved to her front end. We waited for five more minutes to be sure that the drug had worked, and John asked if we could move in. It seemed okay, so we made a routine sweep close to the group to ensure she was not playing possum before we landed. The cubs snuggled close to her, right by her head.

Tex settled the helicopter onto the snow on its big, black rubber pontoons, about 100 metres (330 feet) behind the bears. I clambered out with my drug box, ensuring the pistol John had given me was close to hand. John emerged from the seat next to Tex, and we moved off a few paces so we could talk to rather than shout at each other. The noise from the helicopter blade gradually diminished from a roar to a racket as the engine slowed down.

"You go out to the left, pass them by at least 30 metres [98 feet], and get beyond them," John said. "Then, start to

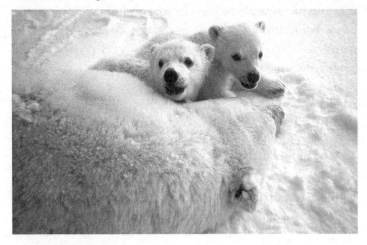

Close to mum is best

circle back slowly and drop to your knees as you come in. Crawl the last 20 metres [65 feet] or so. Take your cue from me. This is how we get in close and not scare off the cubs by being above them."

As I turned away, he continued, "Make sure you have that gun loaded and ready. I will be doing the same on the other side and won't be ahead of you with my rifle." With his story of Ray's close encounter fresh in my head, I hardly needed reminding, but appreciated the emphasis on safety.

As part of his basic safety drill, when still 15 metres (50 feet) away from the bears, John balled up a mitt full of snow and lobbed it at the bear's head, missing by a good 20 centimetres (8 inches). His next effort was on the mark and bounced off her black nose. No response. He edged closer, to about 5 metres (15 feet) and tried again. Still no reaction to the direct hit.

Meanwhile, I was watching the rise and fall of her chest, which was slow but steady. She was breathing four times a minute. We moved in, and I drew up tiny doses of the mixture for the cubs, which looked about half as big as my black Labrador at home. It was easy to inject them in the rump; they looked back at me but offered no aggression. They were out cold in a few minutes.

Ray, John and I had discussed the protocol for cubs as small as these on our first day in Pond. Because we knew that the mixture was safe, reliable and easy to administer, we chose it over the super-potent opioid, which was still questionable for use on small cubs.

When the cubs were sedated, John opened his black box with all its tools, and I went through the routine for checking the vital signs of any patient.

❧

CHAPTER 19

Pond Inlet
Part 2: More Work

First, I checked the heart on the female's left side. With my big mitts off I pulled my stethoscope out of the inner pocket of my parka. The first experience of listening to a moose's heart through the earpieces on a cold winter day in Saskatchewan had been a good lesson. Stethoscope earpieces become little more than lumps of artificial ice if they spend any time in an outside pocket, and ice is not a pleasant thing to shove into one's ears.

The bear's heart was beating steadily, the familiar "lub dub" thumping gently away at 44 beats per minute. I shifted the bell up and back to listen to her lungs, which sounded clear and normal. Her breathing rate of four beats per minute seen from a distance seemed to be a false impression. Not so. It was only much later that I found out that carfentanil slows breathing in bears more than in other mammals such as moose, wolves and bison.

The cubs were much easier to listen to; they had heart rates of more than 60 beats per minute, which were appropriate to both the drugging regime and their diminutive size. With the mother stable, I moved back to her rear end and inserted my glass thermometer. I learned many years ago in Africa to tie a length of tape attached to a bulldog clip to the end of the thermometer. It took but a moment to clip it to the ivory-coloured hairs.

If the glass should disappear forward into the opening or drop out and vanish in the snow, it would be inconvenient, to say the least. While the mercury took its standard minute or so to stabilize, I checked her heart again. It was standard procedure to check vitals every five minutes during the next 40 minutes until we had finished our work.

Tex had moved his machine up closer to the worksite, which would help when we finished up and the mother bear got her injection of antidote.

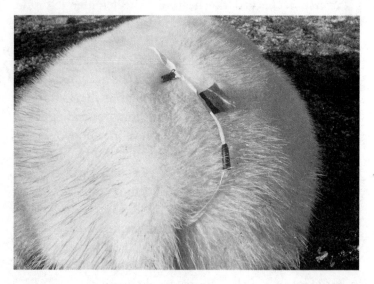

A bulldog clip prevents awkward moments.

While I checked the vital signs, John took out a pair of tattooing pliers and inserted a new number that would be a permanent record. He opened up a toothpaste-like tube and squeezed out a length of green goop, which he applied to the inside of the animal's lip with his index finger. Then he placed the pliers over the dye and squeezed hard. With the pliers back in the box, he put his finger under the lip again and rubbed hard for several seconds. Finally he turned the lip up to check that the numbers were visible. These numbers would mark the bear for the rest of her life. The process is the same as that used to tattoo registered puppies, although dogs get theirs in the earflap. Should she be captured again in subsequent years, her permanent record could be found. Researchers, even other teams, would know where she was first caught and how far from there she had moved.

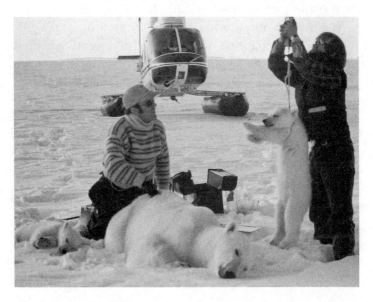

Weighing time for a cub

Then it was time to weigh the bears. For the cubs, it was easy. John put them in a sling and hung them up on a luggage scale.

As for the mother bear, we used a flexible measuring tape that looks much like the ones a tailor uses but is designed for weighing cattle. We slid it under and around her chest at armpit level and read off the numbers.

The measurements were initially verified using tripods and scales, but that is more time-consuming and cumbersome than using a length of tape that can be rolled up and put in the corner of a toolbox. (Later work showed that this tape-measuring technique is not accurate in bears.) The number was recorded on two data sheets. I had developed the boilerplate for my data sheet over many years and many types of patients. John, too, had his own version, and although his was set up differently, the information we recorded was virtually identical.

As I carried out another all-round check of vital signs, John got two small, white ear tags with a number etched

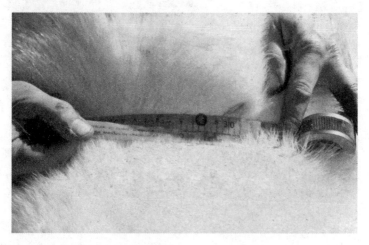

A tape measure to gauge weight

on them and punched them into the mother's ears. We rolled the bear onto her back and took a blood sample from the big vein in her inner thigh, where the hair is much less dense than on the neck, making it a better spot to draw blood than from the jugular. I didn't put the tubes of blood into my box because they would surely freeze over the course of the day. Instead, I slipped them under my parka and into the old cummerbund that my wife Jo had adapted by adding pockets. My favourite aunt had given me the cummerbund for my 21st birthday. It was a bit ragged, long past its prime as a fashion accessory with a tuxedo. I don't even know why I kept it. Nostalgia maybe? But, surely neither my aunt nor my 21-year-old self could have foreseen its transition into a research tool.

The bear's temperature had risen by less than half a degree, and all else seemed well. I took a small fecal sample in a plastic glove turned inside out. The sealed glove went into a Whirl-Pak® sample bag and, along with the small card with the bear's tattoo number, was packed into the black box.

With a pair of pliers, John plucked a bunch of hair from the back of her neck and dropped it with another card into a sample bag. The hair would be analyzed for its chemical makeup and any contaminants in the environment that had been absorbed by the bear.

John drew out another pair of pliers, dental extractors for very small teeth, and a third sample bag. Just behind the big canine tooth that is part flesh-tearing tool and part weapon is a tiny vestigial tooth. It has no function in the bear's life, but for the researcher it is invaluable because it can be sliced and studied under a microscope in the lab. Just as the growth rings in a tree reveal its age, so the rings in this premolar tell the age of the bear. Age information gathered about a bear population reveals whether not bears are being overhunted. If the population contains the appropriate ratio of young to old bears, it can sustain hunting. Of course, polar bear hunting is extremely important to the Inuit people, but overhunting needs to be guarded against. This information was an important component of the research we were doing at the time.

Next came the last mucky task. John brought out a tube of black Lady Clairol© hair dye and a brush. Before long, a huge black X, each arm about 60 centimetres (24 inches) long, followed by a number covered the bear's back from side to side. John explained the reason for applying the dye was to ensure that any bear we dealt with would not be captured again that year. The "X" indicated that the bear was captured in Canada; bears in other regions carried a different letter.

There was no need to paint the cubs because they would be with their mother for two more years. I wonder if the folks at Clairol ever imagined such a use for their product.

I made the rounds with the stethoscope again, and John read off his checklist to ensure that we had not forgotten a vital element. Once the final check was complete, we hunkered down to wait for the cubs to recover. We didn't have to wait for the mother to come out of it because I could give her the antidote to the carfentanil. Not so for the drugs used for the cubs. And we couldn't wake the mother until the little guys were alert, but that didn't take long. In fact, by the time we had wrapped up our duties, they were already showing signs of recovery, moving their tongues and heads as we finished collecting our various samples. From that point, their recovery was rapid, and they soon snuggled up to their mother.

Ten minutes later I drew up the antidote and injected it into the vein on the underside of her tongue, which was easy to get at. We had already packed up our gear because neither of us wanted to be fiddling with it when the bear awoke, as she would do within three or four minutes.

Tex started up the helicopter engines on John's signal because he needed time to get his machine revved up and airborne. Again, should my patient decide to come after us, we wanted to be up and away before she reached us. A bear can cover a lot of ground very quickly if it wants to.

We walked as briskly back to the chopper as the deep snow would allow, rather than run and risk falling. Tex upped the revs, lifted off, backed a safe distance away and

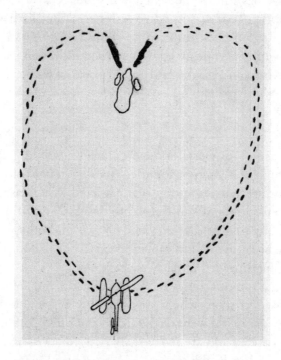

Sketch of the aerial view for an approach to an immobilized bear. The solid marks near the bears represent the close approach when workers are crawling to reduce profile.

hovered for a short while. The bear rose, stumbled once and moved away with her little cubs alongside her.

With the work on these bears complete, Tex climbed above the site and looked down. Our tracks in the snow and the helicopter landing spot resembled the shape of a Valentine's Day heart. Earlier researchers had worked out the pattern when approaching mothers and cubs. The drawback is that one cannot be absolutely sure the mother is really immobilized, so any team is always crawling up to a potential mauling.

As we flew off in the helicopter, I looked over to where the mother bear was walking with her cubs. The hair-dye marker stood out clearly, so we could avoid harassing her again while still noting how far she had moved. It was time to move on and maybe find another bear, if we were lucky.

It was not all work. Some evenings we would gather at the home of a young Mountie. His wife's circle of friends had formed a social group that gathered weekly as a photography club and had learned to develop and print their work. She told us that they had chosen photography over bridge because the card game tended to be too competitive and sometimes led to nasty exchanges.

After a fun but somewhat shambolic game of softball on the town airstrip, which was the only place sufficiently clear of snow, we went to the local (and only) coffee shop.

I am sort of addicted to Mars Bars, a situation that stems from a 12-year-old schoolboy visit to the Mars factory near my school. The only place I thought I might find one in Pond was at the Co-op store, so I headed there. I was

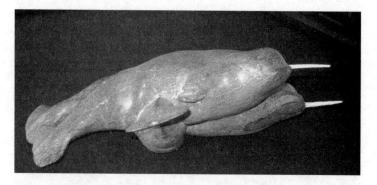

Joanasee Simonee's soapstone carving of narwhal at play

able to fill my comfort-food needs for five days (one a day; you must not overdo these things).

A soapstone carving caught my eye. It was a beautiful, grey-green soapstone carving of three narwhal, created by Joanasee Simonee, the school janitor. Eventually, it became hand luggage.

The next day we went out again with Ray up beside Tex and John behind. I was seated behind Tex in case we had a chance to do some darting. He and I needed to be on the same side of the aircraft so that we could coordinate. Within 15 minutes, as we crested a rise over a small ridge, we saw a big bear at a dark spot on the ice. A muddled mass of incoming tracks toward what was soon evident as a carcass beside a hole showed clearly in the snow. Many footprints were around the hole where a seal had been caught and partially eaten.

The bear was heading away but hadn't gone more than 50 metres (165 feet) when we dropped down. We soon had him darted and processed. The most interesting thing about him was the state of his teeth and the scars on his face. Two of his big canines were snapped off, the left one near the gum line. He had obviously been in more than

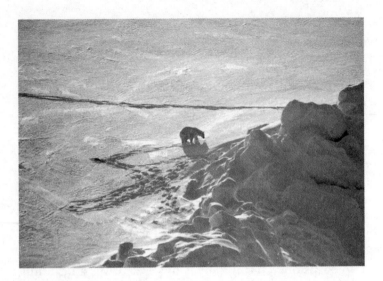

A big male leaving a seal hole

one fight. I've seen the same thing in free-ranging lions in Africa. I walked back to the seal hole to take a look.

The only remnants of the seal were a partly chewed jaw-bone and some scraps of hair. Beside the hole were small footprints of what must have been a fox. There were also prints of some largish bird. John explained that they were raven prints.

"They often show up at a kill site to clean up the scraps," he said.

Ten days later we had accomplished everything Ray had planned. It was time to go home, and my main challenge was to work out the best way to pack my purchase.

An Upset Elk

This fire needed instant attention before it proved fatal.

One of the simplest and at the same time most dangerous "fires" in the zoo occurred when the resident bull elk decided to take out his frustrations on the braided cable that kept him from destroying the page-wire fence separating him from the viewing public. Before the cable was added, the fence sagged like an old skirt.

In early September he began to rut. Over the next week or so his fervour became full-blown. With his neck stretched out and his prepuce moving backward and forward, he let rip with a series of blood curdling, high-pitched sounds that echoed like a trumpet with a sore throat. What the folks living in the houses outside the zoo perimeter thought has not been recorded, but I'm sure small children got the willies and nervous maiden aunts were kept awake in the night. The sound was meant to show any other elk within earshot who was boss. That no potential rivals lived within 100 kilometres (60 miles) didn't stop him for a moment. But as we arrived each morning, the sound was a reminder to those working at the zoo that all was well with the world.

As his ardour grew more furious, the palpitations of his prepuce turned into outright thrashing. As he thrashed, he spewed a stream of pungent urine that sprayed forward onto the long black hairs under his neck. It also ended up on the clothing of any visitor unwise enough to stand too close to the fence. The fluid has powerful scent-bearing chemicals not present at other times, with a distinctive smell that is intended to attract females. Every now and then he attacked just about anything whether it moved or not, except of course, his harem.

As any wildlife observer knows, these attacks in the wild are often directed towards shrubs and trees. In the zoo none were available, so almost anything would do as a substitute. But had he succeeded in breaching the page wire, who knows what might have happened.

On one of these days, Stu appeared in my office in a state. Between puffs and pants he told me that he needed my help at the elk pen in a hurry. We loaded the van as quickly as we could with the dart gun, the blowgun, ropes and drugs.

He explained, "The big bull has attacked that thick cable in his pen. He has managed to twist his antler into it. He can't get free."

On a more detailed look, it was clear why the bull could not extricate himself. The cable was wrapped around the long axis of his right antler as well as around one of the seven smaller branched tines. Obviously exhausted but highly frustrated, he was struggling to escape. He could probably not take much more without doing himself serious harm, not so much from direct damage to his body, but from overexertion.

Stu came up with the solution in a split-second. Before we had time to reason out the risks, we were over the fence and grappling with the cable. I untangled the antler in a counter-clockwise fashion while Stu twisted the cable clockwise. We had it done in less than a minute. Then came the tricky part— avoid getting skewered.

The bull was either grateful for our intervention (unlikely) or keen to get back to his "wives." He trotted off to the other side of the enclosure, and we escaped by clambering over the fence.

CHAPTER 20

A Scary Night

In August 1982 I returned to the Arctic only four months after that first trip. This time it was to the Clyde River, about halfway along the northeastern shore of Baffin Island. The river feeds into a fjord, one of dozens that cut into the island's coastline like giant jagged tooth roots.

One thing had me worried after our trip to the Pond Inlet area. Ray and John used a hand-held syringe to inject yearling bears. This technique was fine for tiny cubs, but a frightened yearling or a two-year-old was a different matter. Wrenching a hand away from snapping jaws seemed far too dangerous.

Using the blowgun from a short distance away would reduce the risk. The only problem was that the airport security folks might be alarmed by the metre-long (3-foot) piece of plastic pipe with a mouthpiece at one end. However, all I needed to manufacture the darts was a hacksaw, some hypodermic needles and a length of wool. For the barrel, I substituted a length of half-inch copper pipe, as found at almost any hardware store in Canada. To create a mouthpiece all I needed was a syringe case, the hacksaw and some tape.

On this trip, we were in for a few surprises, some not as nice as others. The first surprise occurred at the wooden shed that served as the arrival and departure hall. One of my two pieces of luggage had not arrived. Unfortunately, it was the pack crammed with winter clothing and gear ranging from underpants to wool socks, long johns, sweaters and wool shirts, as well as my sleeping bag. This was not a happy situation. But because they were too bulky to pack I had worn my parka, wind-proof mittens, hoodie, toque, heavy wool khaki trousers and felt-lined, canvas winter boots. I was lucky, I suppose, to have those items, although they didn't exactly make a fashion statement.

Fortunately, I had carried the immobilizing drugs on board rather than consigning them to a freezing luggage compartment and the possible interest of any unscrupulous baggage handlers. That lot was likely worth hundreds of thousands of dollars to anyone trading in narcotics.

My dark mood quickly brightened when Bob Wooley, the government wildlife officer in the community solved the clothing problem. We were about the same size, and he at once offered to lend me any clothes I might need, even an unopened packet of underwear.

Bob also proved to be a talented musician. That evening as we sipped a beer, he took out his guitar and played some humorous pieces he had composed as well as more traditional songs we all knew. The one I recall most vividly was about the relationship of a male with his penis, from vibrant youth to the fading days of erectile dysfunction.

His tenor voice rang clear as he started with a four-line verse:

> *There are songs that must be sung and there are words that*
> *must be said,*
> *for there's things that leave you sleepless when you lay at night*
> *in bed.*
> *And that's why I sing this song to you and I hope you under*
> *stand*
> *When I sing about the love between a young boy and his hand!*

The next day, Bob had no trouble finding the necessary copper pipe in his office store. In less than 10 minutes the blowgun was ready, with syringe case and tape attached. We even had a little competition with some target practice using a piece of cardboard propped against the wall. I had lots of experience, whereas the others were new to the game. The outcome was definitely one-sided.

With a new pilot, who I will call Andrew, we carried on more-or-less where we had left off near Pond Inlet. The summer melting had left less sea ice, so we could continue our work and also capture a few bears on land.

It did not take long, usually less than five minutes, for a bear to progress from staggering to sitting then lying stretched out. From that point we could easily do all the routine things on our checklists.

Another surprise was the bear with a fresh cut low down on his left hind leg. We had never seen one like it before and did not ever again. He was a juvenile male, perhaps a three-year-old. The good thing was that there were no severed tendons. We speculated on a possible cause, but came up with no sensible idea. We all agreed, however, that it was unlikely to be the result of a fight. Maybe the bear had had an accident with some discarded piece of

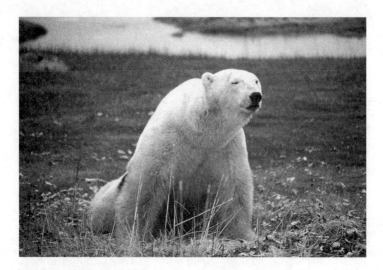

Nearly down and out

garbage. I gave him an injection of antibiotic, sprayed the wound with a bright purple disinfectant and hoped he would make it.

Two days later came another surprise—this time a scary one that might have had severe consequences for all of us. Andrew had forgotten to pack the fuel pump in the cargo hold, a cardinal sin for a helicopter pilot. Being stranded 70 kilometres (43 miles) down the Baffin coast could be fatal. There we were, the fuel gauge reading almost empty and no way to top up from the 165-litre (44-gallon) drums that had been left expressly for our use.

We were not impressed. Siphoning was not an option because the top of the barrel was below the level of the chopper's fuel intake. In addition, the proper method of refuelling involved the filter, which is part of the pump assembly.

Andrew seemed less concerned, explaining that part of his training, and indeed the aircraft certification, involved the process of autorotation. I can't explain the physics, but

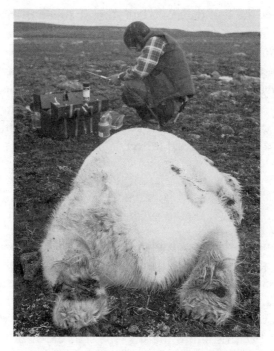

As we work on land, John examines an injured foot.

it sounded as if it had something to do with reversed air-flow through the rotating blades. He seemed confident, so we set off back toward base.

We flew high enough above the land to ensure that the rotors would rotate without power. I was certain we were flying on fumes by the time the community 20 kilometres (12 miles) across the estuary came into view. Unfortunately, the estuary had still not frozen. Andrew calmly told us that there was no way he was going across to the other side and run the risk of autorotating onto a wet surface. We landed near the cliff top and made a radio call to the base. Luckily they picked up the signal but told us that it would be three or four hours before they could get to us.

It was the half dark of a late August Arctic night, a few days after the end of the 24 hours of daylight period. It was too cold to just sit around waiting for rescue, so we put up the emergency tent and broke out two heavy-duty sleeping bags. We took turns guarding the chopper and ourselves. I took first shift, fully dressed in my own and borrowed cold weather gear. Andrew took a rifle from its hard case and passed it over.

~

Sitting on the black rubber floats of a downed helicopter on a frigid Arctic night, rifle cradled across your lap, makes you feel tiny and inconsequential in the landscape of dark rocks and white lumps. The sky arches all the way overhead. A sliver of new moon, seemingly no thicker than an orange peel, rises into the sky. The stars are as brilliant as you have ever seen them because there is no light pollution from any source. It is absolutely still and silent; even the wind has died down. The vague outline of a tent 30 metres (98 feet) away is the only unnatural object. You know it's a tent, but it looks like just another lump of rock.

In this place, under these spooky conditions, humans are not at the top of the food chain. Inuit hunters say that if a bear shows up, it is best to decamp at once. Tex, the pilot who flew the previous trip, mentioned that bears have been known to rip out the bubble of a helicopter with a single swipe.

Suddenly, something white moved at the ten o'clock position, about 100 metres (330 feet) away. I raised the rifle, finger on the trigger, and peered through the scope. The scene cleared at once. The big snow-covered rock was not moving and has not for hundreds, if not thousands, of years. It was a hair-on-the-back-of-the-neck-standing-up moment, and not the last one that night. This strange phenomenon happened five times in the hour and a half shift before I woke the others and crashed asleep almost before the zip on the sleeping bag had reached its top.

Several African folk stories tell of animal transformations, but to me these seem to be more scared false impressions than anything else. Later, I learned that African tales are not the only stories that involve shapeshifting.

In an interview with Inuit elder Aipilik Innuksuk, John MacDonald, who managed the Igloolik Research Centre for the Nunavut Research Institute, learned that transformations by bears are not considered unusual.

In answer to one of John's questions, Innuksuk replied: "Yes, when they don't want to be caught I have experienced bears turning into other things such as birds, foxes, or even ice."

These beliefs are testament to the huge importance of polar bears in Inuit life. I wondered if my impressions of bears approaching me as I sat exposed on the helicopter floats were of a similar nature.

My time on that unusual rubber seat was not entirely taken up with worry about bears. I am fascinated by the stars and have no trouble recognizing the great bear or Orion and his belt. The Seven Sisters, more scientifically known as the Pleiades (the name derived from Greek mythology) are not far from Orion's shoulder. That night I saw them low in the sky off to my right.

In the '90s, MacDonald lived many years in Igloolik, which is only one degree of latitude south of Clyde, but a seven-hour flight west. He wrote the book *The Arctic Sky*. In his fascinating and detailed text, full of helpful diagrams and beautiful photographs, he wrote that polar bears appear in many Arctic legends and are frequently referred to in descriptions of star clusters and constellations. He recorded:

> *The Pleiades were for Inuit an important and widely recognized star cluster. The names given to this cluster by various Inuit groups reflect, to some extent, the role played by the Pleiades in their legends. Frequently the cluster is said to represent a bear surrounded by baying dogs.*

He recorded 24 different names for the Pleiades across the Arctic from Alaska to Greenland. There are also several references to polar bears in other constellations that he discusses in his book.

Researchers have a couple of theories about the bubble destruction behaviour of bears. Andrew Derocher, a long-term polar bear researcher thinks that the bears love to play with the Plexiglas® and has witnessed two such "games" at Churchill.

Dr. Susan Blum gave a slightly different explanation. She worked for six years as a researcher in the High Arctic and at Churchill, earning a PhD for her work. She then held the post of Polar Bear Biologist for the government of Nunavut before moving to Saskatoon. Her chopper bubble account stems from the time when she was working out of Cape Churchill. Her pilot, Steve Miller, thought that the bears would see their reflection in the Plexiglas® and then bash it in. He also told her that the bears would tear out the seats and chew on them. They did the same to the quad bikes, and as a result, the bikes had to be kept inside the fence at the camp.

Either way, polar bears are seriously strong. Susan also recounted an event that gives further evidence of the bear's power. After a huge storm blew in from Baffin Bay into

Lancaster Sound, she saw some beluga whales and one young bowhead whale trapped in a small area of open water, called a *savsaat* by the Inuit. It was surrounded by vast expanses of thick ice so the whales had no hope of reaching the open sea. A big male bear jumped on top of a beluga, and then blood clouded the water.

She did not see the bear haul the whale out, but when the team went back the next day, the carcass was on the sea ice by the *savsaat*. That's pretty strong circumstantial evidence. Any other explanation would be preposterous. The bear probably drowned the whale by submerging

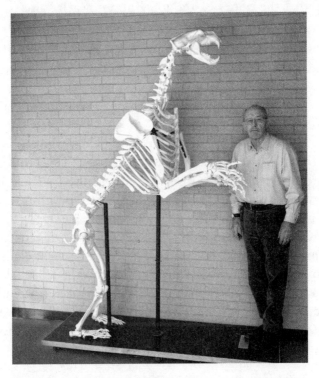

The polar bear skeleton, dedicated to the late Dr. Malcolm Ramsay, at the Western College of Veterinary Medicine

it—powerful stuff. An adult male whale weighs about 1500 kilos (3300 pounds); adult females weigh somewhat less. In human terms a seriously strong man can lift about two and half times his own weight. The bear-to-whale ratio in this case is about the same, but probably involves the use of only one arm. Quite a feat!

As Sherlock Holmes said, When you have eliminated the impossible, whatever remains, however improbable, must be the truth.

Looking at the skeleton of a huge male bear in the atrium of the veterinary college in Saskatoon it is easy to see that the bones of the forearm are heavier and more robust than those of the upper arm. Had it been a bear rather than a wolf in the Red Riding Hood story, it might have been "All the better to grab you with, my dear."

The fuel arrived as promised. Two men came across the fiord in a 5-metre (16-foot) aluminum boat and carried the fuel and pump up the steep cliff in red plastic 15 litre (4-gallon) jerry cans to our stranded chopper.

With that memorable and scary night at an end, we continued to work on bears for a few more days. On the way home, after 16 days away, I went to the left luggage department at the Montreal airport. My green backpack, properly identified, and even showing the tags for delivery to Clyde River was right there, waiting patiently for me.

An Outbreak and a Remedy

Two days before my family headed out on a canoe trip, Gerhard found a dead elk calf in the middle of the enclosure. It looked as if it had some diarrhea before dying. We sent the carcass to the vet college as part of the now well-established routine of taking any animal that died on the zoo grounds to the postmortem room.

Five days later, with memories of a great trip, breadcrumb-coated fried walleye and beautiful sunsets, we headed home to put a nice catch of northern pike and walleye in the freezer. Monday morning, and it was time to head back to the office. It was evident immediately that the situation at the zoo had become more serious. Three more animals, two goats and a donkey, had died. All showed the same signs postmortem, mainly inflamed intestines.

Samples from the animals had immediately been sent upstairs to the bacteriology lab. Within a day they had all grown identical colonies of bacteria. The presumptive diagnosis of Salmonellosis was reasonable, but we needed confirmation, which would take a few more days. At that stage in the science of bacteriology, four days was reasonable. Final confirmation of the specific type *Salmonella* (or any other bacterial infection) would take another four weeks. Today, with the use of the DNA-based polymerase chain reaction (PCR), the complete process can be accomplished in four hours.

Within a week the death toll had risen to nine animals, all fitting the same profile.

It was in his classic 1959 story *Goldfinger* that Ian Fleming had Bond state: "Once is happenstance, twice is coincidence, three times is enemy action."

Nine is way more than three.

A careful search revealed three dead sparrows in the feed bins: two more in the elk pen and one in the bison pen provided the final clues. The latest casualties brought the total number of animal deaths (sparrows included) to 12. Bacterial cultures from the birds taken at the college showed the same results as the mammals that had died.

By mid-week all the animals were started on a course of anti-biotics. No more animals died, so either the treatment worked or the situation had run its course.

The *Salmonella* family of bacteria is well known to cause food poisoning in humans all over the world. It is usually food-borne and is often associated with improper food handling in restaurants. Radio and television report outbreaks fairly frequently. A recent report from Australia described nearly 1900 cases of the disease.

The "closest-to-home" outbreak among my zoo colleagues occurred after a banquet held during the 1996 convention of the American Association of Zoo Veterinarians in Puerto Vallarta, Mexico. One third of the 454 folks who attended came down with diarrhea and other unpleasant symptoms. Some were severely ill and had to be put on intravenous drips. All the cases were linked to the chili rellenos served. Luckily I missed the gathering that year.

CHAPTER 21

Return to the Arctic

In May of the following year I returned to the Arctic, this time to Broughton Island (now Qikiqtarjuaq), just off the coast Baffin Island and farther south and east than Clyde River.

While the work differed hardly at all from the two previous trips to Baffin Island, one event sticks in my mind. As we flew over a cliff peak and dropped into the valley below, a big male bear exploded from a cave-like hollow in the snow and ran to shore then into the open water. Ray explained that the hollow was called a summer den and that bears stay there, not feeding or carrying out any bodily functions that would require the burning of energy when no food is available.

"They often hang out in this sort place for the whole summer once the sea ice melts because without ice they cannot hope to find seals to feed on," he explained.

On an off day, when the weather prevented us from flying, I wandered into the tiny Co-op store in the village and found a beautiful sculpture on a dusty shelf. It was a whalebone carving of two beluga whales touching back to belly, front to back. I had no doubt that the animals were belugas. The rounded foreheads and the lack of dorsal fins were the obvious features that identified them. As I wandered round the store, stocked with a few cans of condensed milk, cartons of cigarettes and packets of tea, I kept coming back to the belugas. The shape and flowing form were gorgeous. Anyone with half an imagination could see the white whales touching as they roil in the water, perhaps during mating foreplay. Surely the artist had witnessed such behaviour. The attached tag identified Josespie Kukseak as the artist. The sculpture was marked "NCV," and I asked the young lady behind the counter what those initials meant.

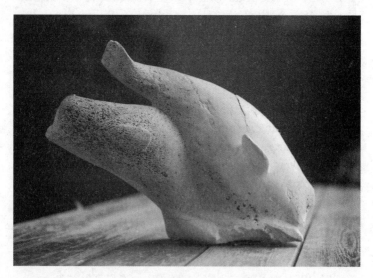

Whalebone belugas at play by sculptor Josespie Kukseak

212

"Oh," she replied, "That means No Commercial Value, so it has been withdrawn from the 'For Sale' shelf." She told me that the NCV label was due to a few longitudinal cracks in the bone that for me in no way detracted from the feeling of play and flowing movement that Mr. Kukseak had portrayed.

Wondering if it was for sale anyway, I asked how much she wanted for it. The cracks did not bother me, and I could not argue with her quote. I had no inclination to haggle. Kukseak had likely created the whales from an old piece of beached whalebone or one taken by traditional hunters and that had eroded over the years. This beautiful object was once again a testament to the life of the Inuit expressed in sculpture, another form of storytelling.

One of my last visits in Broughton was to meet Levi Nutaralak to see how he was progressing with the carving I commissioned the day after I arrived. I met him several times outside his wooden house as he sat and gradually turned a lump of green stone, under his skilled hands, into something he had witnessed. He started with a coarse file. After a few days he switched to a finer one and then to a round one as he began to refine the work. It was a fascinating process to watch. Finally, he spent hours polishing it to create the gorgeous lustre of carved soapstone. He'd created a carving of a bear standing on the body of a dead narwhal. The big carnivore was chewing on its tail flukes. Levi told me that the whale had washed up and died on the beach, and the bear had found it and begun to feed. The beautiful belugas and feeding polar bear artwork live with us to this day.

When the weather cleared, the days were hectic. Some days were much longer than the standard eight- or twelve-hour workday. On the busiest day we kept going for 18 hours straight, tagging 14 bears. Unfortunately sleep

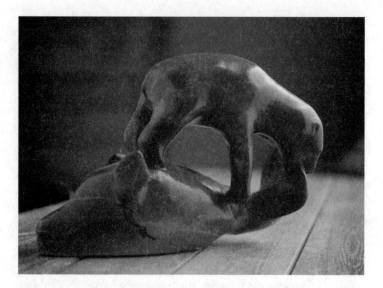

A chance feast for a bear by sculptor Levi Nutaralak

did not come immediately after eating. Ray fell at once into a deep sleep, but John and I still had work to do. An ancient centrifuge sat on the small table in our room. A steady turn with a crank handle generated the spin, but it could hold only four test tubes at a time. We had to spin three tubes of blood collected from each bear in order to extract the serum that I would take back to the lab in Saskatoon for testing. Finally, each tube had to be labelled and frozen. More than three hours later, we finally collapsed on our beds and fell into a coma.

While our immobilization results were encouraging, we still had one hurdle to leap. The carfentanil that we had used on the 63 bears at Pond Inlet, Clyde River and Broughton Island was impossible for a biologist who was not a vet to obtain or use. As a super-potent member of the opioid group, which includes morphine, heroin and several other drugs, carfentanil is tightly restricted. With all the bear work going on in Canada and the U.S., as well as several other polar bear studies under way across the north, another drug was needed.

Several researchers, John Lee and Ray Schweinsburg among them, asked why a drug called Telazol had not been tried in bears. Plenty of literature recorded this drug's use in other species, mainly in zoos, and in some other carnivores, but not a word about bears.

I thought about this issue while heading home but not to the exclusion of other weighty matters. I had been able to snag a few Arctic char in the 2- to 5-kilogram (4.5- to 11-pound) range and had them frozen and packed in a box labelled "samples." The hotel in Montreal had willingly agreed to put my package in their big freezer along with the two others that did indeed contain blood samples from the bears. We had some delicious meals at home that winter—of char, that is, not bear blood.

Once I settled down in Saskatoon, the Telazol question surfaced again. It seemed strange that it had never been reported as being used in any bear research.

There is no harm in trying to make your own luck. This situation seemed to be an opportunity to have a go at changing the scene and making my own luck.

Almost on a whim, even after my veterinary colleagues in the zoo world told me it would be a waste of time, I wrote to the Warner Lambert Company, pitching not only my experience but also the charismatic status of polar bears and our search for safer and surer ways to immobilize them. The response, in the pre-internet days of 1983, surprised me by both its speed and positive nature. The writer was delighted to be of help and would ship samples of the drug to the college pharmacy right away. That protocol, rather than shipping directly to me was needed to make the transfer legal. I did not want to be labelled or arrested as a drug dealer.

The same day as the letter arrived, I mentioned my correspondence to a biology student friend named Malcolm Ramsay as we sat waiting for a graduate class seminar to start. The subject of the course was Advanced Reproductive Physiology. I was working towards a master's degree on the seasonality of reproduction in North American elk, while Malcolm was pursuing loftier goals towards a PhD along the same line but with polar bears instead of elk. Malcolm, with his gravelly voice, goatee beard and floor-mop-like unruly shock of prematurely salt-and-pepper hair was at once interested.

"How soon will you be able to get some," he asked.

"Why?" I replied. "What did you have in mind?"

He pushed his thick-lensed glasses up his nose and told me he was working with Ian Stirling at Churchill and that they would be going to the field in the fall, about six months hence. "I'm interested because we are down to our last few vials of Sernylan. We've heard about Telazol but can't get it. Why don't you call Ian?"

I acted on his idea and was at once invited to join the team at Churchill. Little did I realize what was in store and what a complex character I would meet.

Before long, with the usual paperwork done, I had enough Telazol to hopefully capture at least 60 bears. My first task was to find out if Telazol worked and if it was safe for bears. We had no polar bears at the zoo, but I figured that our black bears would be a place to start. Once again, the two cubs that had arrived in spring were to be euthanized after the school children had visited on Labour Day at the beginning of September. This practice that I wrote about in Chapter 14 still disturbed me, but at least I had a perfect opportunity to gain some useful knowledge.

I knew that Telazol had been used in a variety of other species, especially carnivores. However, safety was a concern because in a couple of reports of its use in tigers, the big cats had died, and nobody had quite worked out why. Luckily my supply of drugs had arrived well before the black bear cubs were due to be euthanized.

I followed my self-imposed rule of first testing any new product on just one animal, in case some unforeseen problem occurred. So I used it at the dose reported for several other species. It worked well. The cub was down and out in just over three minutes and recovered fully 90 minutes later. At a slightly higher dose in the other cub all went well. On the day that the bears were to meet their ends, I tested the Telazol again. Things again went smoothly. Four out of four was at least a strong positive indication, if not absolute proof.

After the tests, I was only slightly worried about the efficacy on polar bears. I began to pack for the October trip.

CHAPTER 22

Déjà Vu on an Unusual Lion Case

E arly in 2015, Lesley Avant, who had been with the Saskatoon Zoo Society as a member and then employee for over 30 years, forwarded an email to me. A 14-year-old boy in Winnipeg explained how he had been told stories by his granddad about a lion.

Zachary wrote: "He used to be a professor of dentistry at the University of Saskatchewan during the '70s and '80s. He always used to tell me how you came to him seeking his help to make the world's first set of dentures for a lion."

That was not quite how I recalled the case, but I have the advantage of a set of photos taken that day and a short article I wrote for the *Journal of Zoo Animal Medicine* (as it was called in those days).

~

When the keepers told me that George was off his feed, and had only been toying with the chunks of meat and bone over the last couple of days, it was obvious that we needed to do something. To immobilize him, we tricked the old lion. I went over to this pen, so as usual, he promptly headed to the other side, as far away from me as possible. He had obviously forgotten that his conditioned reaction would not always mean safety from injections. Stu used the blowgun with the typical accuracy of an experienced hunter to get a drug cocktail into him. George turned and snarled, but it was too late.

Within a few minutes, he was out cold. Sharon poked at him with a long stick through the wire. No reaction. It was an encouraging sign. We could now enter his pen because Queenie, the lioness, was safely locked in the shelter.

I measured his vitals; his heart and breathing were normal. Next I put some drops into his eyes to protect them from dust, and only then did I look at his mouth.

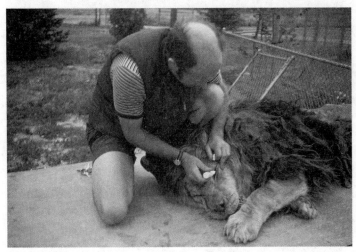

Eye drops for a lion

It was easy to see what the problem was. He had three broken canine teeth, the big ones that a lion uses to kill his prey. Two of them had nasty-looking pus-like material oozing out. No wonder he was off his feed. He must have been in pain.

The situation was beyond my skills; I needed help. By lunchtime I was back in my office at the veterinary college and on the phone to the dental college across campus. Two mornings later we were back at the zoo, and by we, I mean four dentists and me. Four was almost certainly three more dentists than we actually needed, but it's not every day a chance like this came along. Indeed, one of the dentists told his grandson about the case some 35 years later.

Immobilization was much easier this time because the keeper staff had shut Queenie out of the shelter, and George was within easy reach for his injection.

The dental team made an impression cast of George's mouth. As the cast dried, they discussed an idea for making up a set of metal crowns.

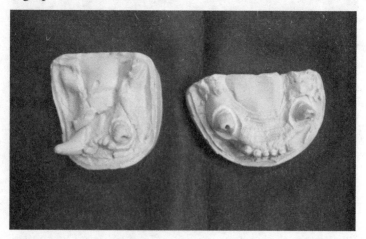

Not quite a normal tooth impression cast

We discussed the possibilities of how George had broken his teeth. I had seen broken teeth in wild lions and had learned that they were usually the result of fights—obviously not the case in George's situation. His broken teeth were likely the result of him biting at the wires around his cage and catching the rear, concave surfaces of his teeth. When he pulled back they got stuck and broke off, a recognized hazard for lions in captivity.

Our third immobilization, for a much longer procedure, took place a few days later. Again, George was easy to approach in his shelter, and the routines were simple.

We carried him to a waiting flatbed trailer where I again administered eye drops and put a towel over his head. We then shifted the sleepy lion into the zoo van and headed to the college. Once we arrived, the anesthesia team led by

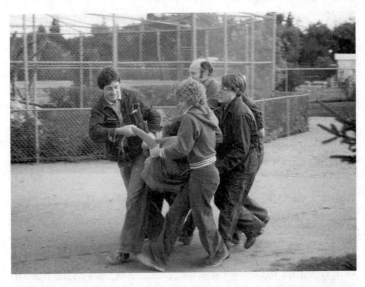

Lifting George out of his pen and off to the trailer. Clockwise from left: Stu Hampton, author, two unnamed students, Sharon Latour (later Schmitt).

221

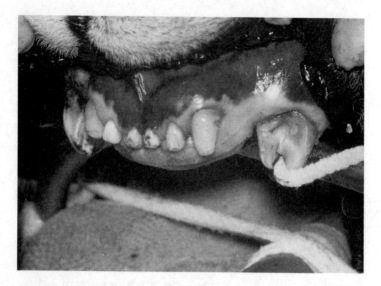

Before: pipe cleaners have more than one use.

Peter Cribb joined us. These folks would have to keep both George and the teams safe for a couple of hours. We did not want him waking up mid-surgery!

At this point I was more-or-less redundant. The dentists took over for the root canals on not just one tooth, but on three. They had come fully prepared. None of their usual delicate instruments was going to be of much use, but of course, all necessary equipment had to be autoclaved. What the technician in the sterilizing suite thought of the weird collection has not been recorded. To clean out the infected tooth roots, they used coping saw blades that they'd picked up at a hardware store. Flushing the mess out of the root canals was easier. Instead of their normal fine equipment, they used large needles, and there was no shortage of those around. To dry everything, they had sterilized a whole bunch of pipe cleaners.

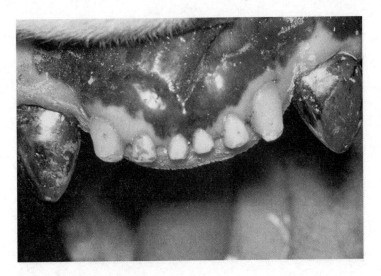

After: George's new teeth.

Then came the really clever bit: the dentists had designed stainless steel tooth caps that had no concave surfaces. With the canals and teeth dry and clean, it was simply a case of applying the right sort of cement, albeit in much larger quantities than any human patient needed. They inserted the pins into the channels and let everything dry. If George got at the wires again, the teeth would simply slip off as he pulled.

George soon adapted to his new finery. His appetite returned, and he lived on for quite a few more trouble-free years. During a brief interlude someone thought to rename him Jaws after the nasty fellow played by Richard Dawson Kiel in the James Bond movie *The Spy Who Loved Me*. That didn't last.

George's skull, with teeth in place, is now a part of the collection of bones and other bits in the WCVM's anatomy department.

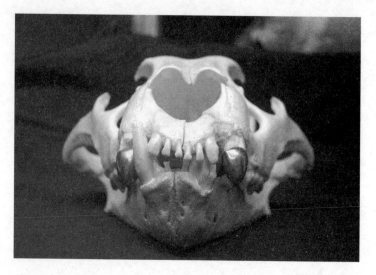

George's skull on display at the Western College of Veterinary Medicine

Every year the vet college students hold a one-day event that is open to the public. The unusual skull appears every now and again in these VetaVision displays. The teeth were never strictly dentures, as Zachary has been told, but at the time they were indeed the world's only set of capped lion's teeth. Perhaps they still are.

CHAPTER 23

Polar Bear Capital
of the World

Over about 40 years, I have made three trips to Churchill at the northern tip of Manitoba, once as a consultant, once as a bear researcher and once as a tourist.

The first was in 1978. It involved a one-hour flight to Winnipeg and a similar one north to Churchill. After our work together on Sable Island, Dr. Harry Rowsell, the interim president of the Canadian Council on Animal Welfare, called to ask if I would be willing to travel to Churchill to evaluate a polar bear research program. Of course I agreed, but that evening I had to dig out our atlas to find Churchill's location. It is on the western shore of Hudson Bay in Manitoba's far north. The town is known as the Polar Bear Capital of the World.

My trip had lasted about a day and a half, with an overnight hotel stop in Churchill, and involved evaluating the health and welfare of a single captive bear being studied by

Norwegian Nils Oritsland and his Canadian graduate student Paul Watts. The two men, along with others, eventually published some important information about several aspects of polar bear physiology.

My memories of the trip are the majestic size and ivory colour of the huge male that Paul had hooked up to monitors. It was sad to see such a magnificent creature in a small cage. I later learned that this sort of temporary confinement has to happen every summer for the safety of both the bears that enter the community and the humans that live there. The alternative is to kill the bears, and nobody is keen on that idea. In 1974, which was a bad year, 147 bears were seen in residential areas of the town. Conservation officers had to kill 11 of them.

My research visit in 1983 at the end of October lasted 10 days longer. We accomplished quite a pile of work with Telazol during that time.

Malcolm was already in town. He picked me up at the airport, and we headed to the Churchill Northern Studies Research Centre, where the team was based. The centre was not the fine building of the same name that exists today, but a much more basic set of somewhat dilapidated single-storey dark brown structures. It was near the airport and across from Akudlik Marsh, famous as the former nesting site of Ross's gulls.

Ian Stirling was the team leader. He had gained his biologist's stripes studying leopard seals in Antarctica. Now he was at the other end of the world studying the most charismatic of all northern species, the polar bear. In 2011 he published an outstanding book that is considered the definitive work on their biology.

The first task the next morning was to visit the hospital. There I told a young doctor what we were doing and gave him information about the Telazol so that he would be prepared for an emergency if an accidental injection occurred.

We worked with other team members during my 10-day stint. Our experienced helicopter pilot was Steve Miller. He had seen the almost unbelievable whale kill when working with Susan Blum. The wildlife technician was Dennis Andriashek, who had worked with Ian for several years and was a crack shot with the dart gun. He did not miss once on more than 30 bears he fired at. The experience was quite unlike my time on Baffin Island.

In 1981, a special facility, known as the "polar bear prison" was built. Bears that enter the townsite are captured and moved there by the staff of the Manitoba Department of Natural Resources, who have been trained in the procedure. Researchers and town residents know the facility as D20.

In some years, there are so many D20 "guests" that they are moved to allow for more. They are immobilized, rolled

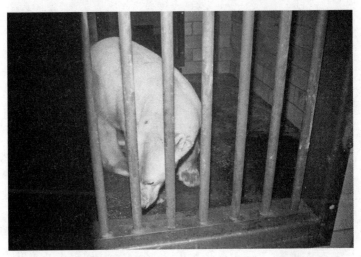

One of several D20 "guests"

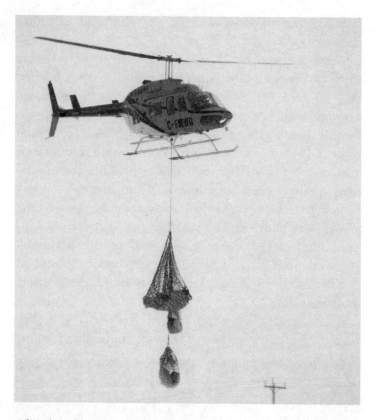

A female and her two cubs leave D20.

into cargo nets and moved at least 80 kilometres (50 miles) from the town before being released. In the fall, once the free-ranging bears have headed back onto the ice, the facility is emptied of its temporary residents.

The new drug needed to be tested one more time on an actual polar bear. D20 was the obvious place to do the testing. We could observe and record everything at close range. All went well, just as it had with the cubs at the zoo. We ended up injecting 11 bears in D20, three of them twice. We also went to the dump, where animals had

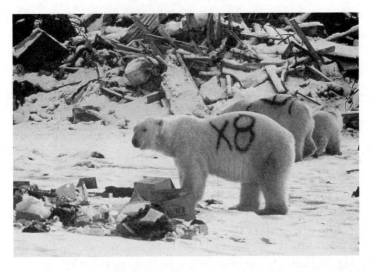

An annual returnee for the free grub. Her yearling cubs were as big as two-year-olds out on the land.

become captive by their stomachs and the abundant food scraps there.

The dump was closed in 2006. This change stopped the bear visits as well as the risks to humans. The town refuse is now stored in an old shipping hub at the town's former military base.

Our first flight for the field study was to the area 20 kilometres (12 miles) east of town to the Hudson Bay Lowlands, (now part of Wapsuk National Park). I was astonished to see a large number of bears so close to the shore. That evening, with the helicopter noise no longer hammering my ears, I asked Ian about this phenomenon.

He explained that every year bears mass along the southern coast of the bay and wait for the sea ice to form so that they can get out to hunt for their main food source, seals, after the long summer of near starvation. While on shore they eat almost nothing.

Malcolm chipped in. "That is the general rule, but occasionally it can be broken," he said. "Do you remember the time we saw a bear sitting on top of a caribou carcass? There were several wolves circling around it, but doing nothing else. At a guess they had killed the caribou, and he had happened to come by at the right moment. He was now obviously telling them, 'This is mine, and you can do nothing about it.'"

As an aside, in 2000, Malcolm and his colleague Dr. Stuart Innes died in a helicopter crash as they returned to Resolute in the Canadian High Arctic after a polar bear tagging day. While polar bear research was Malcolm's main field of study, his interests covered a much wider spectrum. The last time I saw him before he left on that fatal trip, we chatted over tea and doughnuts about possible ways to reduce stress for and improve welfare for the bears.

Working on the open tundra east of Churchill was a completely different kettle of fish from the High Arctic environment of Baffin Island. For a start, we could see little snow, except in sheltered spots on the north-facing side of patches of bush and small creeks. The colours of berries and leaves that remained in a gorgeous array of red, gold and orange was an added visual treat.

As we flew along the shore, we saw several single bears simply lollygagging about. Once or twice pairs or even larger groups of male bears seemed to be hanging out together. On most days one could see as many as a dozen in close proximity. I had little chance to take pictures as we flew along; we were working, not touring. We were on the lookout for lone bears to tag, and I had my hands full of equipment. We did see some females with cubs but never anywhere near males. They stayed well away because, as Ian explained, males tend to prey upon cubs and eat them if they get the chance.

To my great satisfaction, the Telazol worked well in the open tundra for most of the bears. Our routine was straightforward. When we saw an unmarked bear, Ian and I were dropped off, so that the chopper was lighter and safer to maneuver. Steve promptly took off, and within moments brought the chopper down alongside the animal, only a few feet above its head. Almost at once, the machine rocked back slightly and lifted up. We knew that Dennis had fired his dart gun at the bear's neck and shoulder region and had almost certainly hit his mark. We gave each bear time to go down and relax.

"He's good isn't he? Of course, pilot Steve is the real key with darting. He is obviously very experienced. I found this out years ago in Africa. Ninety percent of the success is with the pilot. The gun is easy after that," I said.

"He doesn't often miss," Ian replied.

After about three minutes, the bear staggered and then sat, looking somewhat dazed. Its body slowly subsided until it was lying on its belly, head stretched out. This was pretty standard, just like the cubs I had drugged at the zoo and from many other animals immobilized with a less potent, close relative of Telazol. The last action before full sleep was a licking motion of the tongue. And so it proved.

Finally we started work when the bear did not respond to a pull on his tongue. We had at least an hour to do our work, including ear tagging and lip tattoos.

Steve was more than just a pilot. He was interested and keen on what we were doing and often got involved in the handling process. The bear's tongue began to move as Steve examined him, which meant we still had twenty minutes or so. The return of tongue movement is generally a warning sign of impending recovery, but we soon found that recovery would still take some time. After the tongue

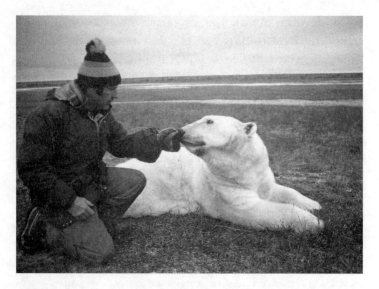

A sniff as the bear regains his faculties

had been moving for a while, the bear's head came up, but he was still "out of it."

From there recovery progressed slowly in reverse, with the bear finally sitting up before it found its feet and wandered away. For a short while it looked like a Friday night drunk.

There were so many bears that on two occasions Dennis took the opportunity to dart two unrelated animals (as opposed to a sow and cubs) within a few minutes and a short distance from one another. And so I had the dubious privilege of attending to two patients at once. The routine was the same as for any other immobilized animal. First, be sure that it was not playing possum. Cover its eyes to protect them then check heart, lungs, pulse and general condition.

I took the stethoscope from my ears, turned from my first tranquilized patient and headed to second one lying just beyond a patch of dwarf birch in a clear spot on the open tundra. It was a trifle unnerving to see another 200-kilogram (440-pound) female ambling ahead across my intended path. The drug box hung from my left hand, and under the other arm, for my own safety, was tucked a double-barrelled shotgun with a single explosive flash shell in one barrel and a slug in the other.

The most important thing to remember was Dennis' warning. "If you have to use the shell when a bear is close, make sure that the explosion and bright flash do not take place on the far side of the bear. This could drive it towards you, rather than away. Not good."

Fortunately, the bear glanced at me and continued on its way. The other team members obviously knew a great deal about bear behaviour at this time of year or they wouldn't have immobilized the second animal or suggested the walk. The gun stayed under my arm.

As I neared the second bear, a big covey of ptarmigan in their all-white winter plumage burst from a patch of bush. On another occasion about 70 of them flew over a big male. Spectacular!

We captured one female because her radio collar needed a new battery. She had two yearling cubs with her. Stirling's team had never seen a blowgun in use, and they were interested. Once again it proved useful for immobilizing the cubs. If I'd gone too close, they could easily have nailed me with those powerful teeth. Not a good idea for any of us; it certainly would have disrupted the workday.

~

I have been involved in collar placement or replacement of several species in Canada and some African countries.

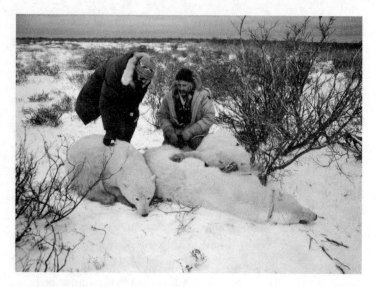

A radio-collared female and her two cubs

Sometimes local people express concerns about effects collars may have on animals.

Inuit elder Aipilik Innuksuk of Igloolik was one such man. In 1995, John Macdonald of the Igloolik Research Centre for the Nunavut Research Institute interviewed him about bears.

I have summarized Mr. Innuksuk's concerns:

> *Bears should not be collared because it will prevent them from hunting successfully. That will lead to a failure to survive. If they cannot survive themselves their cubs will not survive either.*

He further stated that some Inuit had found some of these animals dying because of the tags and collars.

Susan Blum told me that she had heard similar concerns from elders in Arctic communities. She wrote:

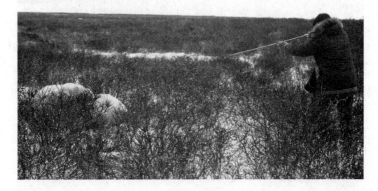

A blowgun is safer than a hand-held syringe for injecting yearlings or two-year-old cubs.

There was no clear evidence of this from the fieldwork that I conducted. Bears with collars had successful pregnancies, healthy cubs and we did not see any difference in weight between bears with collars versus no collars.

My experience has been the same.

~

One bear in particular caught my immediate interest; it was a large emaciated male. The first clue came from Steve. He had observed the animal limping even before approaching it for the shot. As we came up behind, I could see that his left hind leg was bent at an unusual angle. After my routine checks, I lifted the leg and found that the knee could not bend at all.

Ian at once agreed to the suggestion that we try to get the leg x-rayed at the hospital. We were both keen to know what had happened. We had little time to waste because the bear might show signs of waking up, but a top-up dose would simplify the matter.

We had a cargo net in the helicopter baggage compartment, so the four of us rolled him into the net. After we clambered into the seats, Steve lifted off, bear in tow, and took us to the research centre. Our truck was parked near the landing area, and we loaded him into the truck bed for the run to the hospital. The doctor I met that first day gave permission for us to take an X-ray, and because the machine was portable, it could be wheeled to the patient. The truck backed into the garage and the rest was easy. I'm certain that both the doctor and the X-ray technician were seduced by the unusual request and wanted to see a bear up close. They were especially fascinated by the animal's black skin under its ivory-coloured coat.

I lifted the bear's leg up using a short piece of rope attached to a handy bar on the inside of the truck cover and improvised bandages to hold the X-ray plate over the

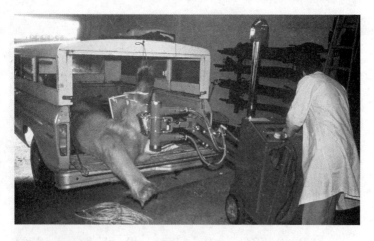

There is a first time for everything—x-raying a bear in a pickup!

knee cap while the machine came up to the right distance and everything was in focus.

Unlike the almost instant digital results of today, in 1983, the plates took time to develop. When we saw the X-ray images, we knew that there was nothing we could do to help. He had been shot, and the knee was a wreck, with fragments of bullet over the remains of the kneecap and a larger bone callus behind it.

By now the patient needed a top-up anesthetic dose. The last thing we needed was for him to wake up in the truck or while unloading him, so we headed back to the tundra.

We could not judge how long his knee had been injured, but because we had found him going about his daily business, we simply watched him until he woke up and meandered away. Like the others we saw, he was waiting for the

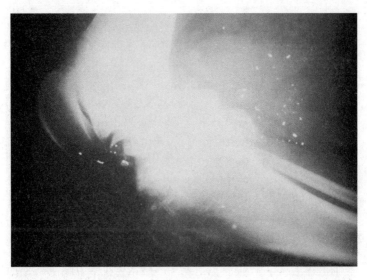

A locked knee with many bone fragments and small pieces of bullet were plain to see.

bay to freeze so that he could get out onto the sea ice to hunt seals and assuage his long summer of near starvation.

In that October 1983, over and above the animals we worked on in D20, we successfully captured 26 more bears without trouble, using just a single dart each time. The objective of a first ever good-sized trial was achieved and gave us a starting place.

Others, including fellow fly-fishing fanatic and former student Nigel Caulkett have refined our initial work and added other useful drugs to make up an effective cocktail for immobilizing bears. The new cocktail of drugs that had not yet been developed in the early 1980s can even be reversed, allowing for a quicker patient wake-up, and not just for polar bears, but for black and grizzly bears as well.

~

My third trip to Churchill in 2014 was with Jo and Paul Sayer, a long-time colleague and good friend from Kenya. We had shared an apartment in our internship years at the vet school at Kabete, not far from Nairobi.

Joining us was Sue Lewis from Vancouver. Not surprisingly Paul's winter gear was borrowed from three of our neighbours, and he still managed to look chilled.

Instead of the two one-hour flights from home I had taken in 1978, we opted for the more "romantic" tourist experience. Our journey north with other like-minded folks involved a five-hour drive in a van, a two-night train ride and a magical trip in a huge, custom-designed polar bear viewing vehicle known as a Tundra Buggy.

The train we took is known as the Muskeg Express. The word "muskeg" derives from the Cree word *maskek* (L⌐ᑫˋ), meaning low-lying marsh. Muskeg is dodgy to drive or

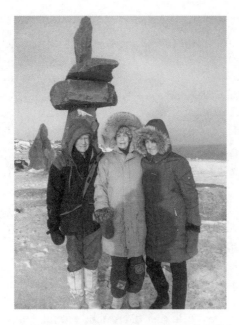

Guess who is the most chilled. From left: Paul, Jo (centre) and Sue.

even walk on in summer when not frozen. The train travels 920 kilometres (570 miles) over muskeg that usually has a water table near its boggy surface. The ride is anything but an express. Indeed it is said that it occasionally moves so slowly that one can overtake it at a walk, but it does run year-round.

The bears were of course the main standout. It was a special feeling to watch them behave without any sense that we might be about to harass them. From the Tundra Buggy we saw 44 in one day. The most spectacular was the big male that examined us as he meandered past a stand of stunted black spruce.

The buggy stopped beside two "teenagers" rolling and play-fighting like a couple of puppies. Although I had seen male bears wrestling 30 years earlier, the other three had

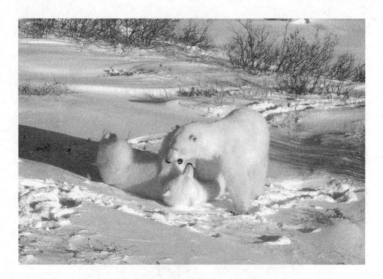

A wrestling match 15 metres (50 feet) from the buggy

not, but it was still just as much a treat for me. After a while, the bears grew tired of the contest and wandered off. Within three minutes, they resumed the fun and games. This time they stood on their hind legs and wrestled rather languidly like a couple of lazy football linemen in training camp or rugby prop forwards in a maul or a lineout. They were not at all aggressive, just goofing around.

Another interesting thing was to watch a bear eating kelp. I wondered if they were after an iodine boost after a long summer lay-off.

When we arrived in Churchill we were unexpectedly delighted by the town's only café. It was obviously used by everyone in town, as well as us tourists. It is called Gipsy's Bakery and Restaurant, owned by long-time residents who hailed from Portugal. After our first visit, I found I needed to return regularly because they serve to-die-for chocolate éclairs. After all, chocolate is one of the essential food

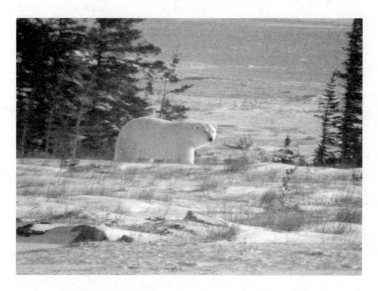

A big male checks us out.

groups. Mixing it with cream simply provides the five-star touch.

I had made three very different trips to Churchill. The first one was a mere taste, a scientific curiosity. The second was a continuation of the free-ranging wildlife studies that have been the backbone and fascination of my career. The third was a delightful opportunity shared with good friends and, of course, with Jo. The trip was intended to be a surprise as a late birthday present and celebration of our engagement 46 years ago to the day. The element of surprise was lost in short order as she queried the large credit card charge that was the deposit for the trip. I had to 'fess up. She enjoyed the trip anyway; the surprise just arrived earlier than I intended.

CHAPTER 24

Rubber Bullet:
A Traumatic Event

While I worked at Churchill with Ian Stirling and his team, my role expanded in an unexpected way. We had just finished a hard day's work south and east of the town when Ian took a call. After he hung up, he turned to me.

"Gord Stenhouse is working over at Cape Churchill as the NWT bear deterrent biologist. He is coming over tomorrow morning with a dead bear. I told him you were here, and he'd like you to do a postmortem."

Of course, I agreed, although I didn't have much in the way of fancy p-m gear, just a good knife, coveralls and a pair of rubber gloves. The missing bits included an apron, scalpel and tweezers, safety glasses and jars of preservative. I also lacked any formal training as a pathologist beyond the basics that stemmed from early days in veterinary school some 20 years earlier and periodic cases that cropped up during my days in Kenya.

Gord brought the carcass to the garage next to the Northern Studies Centre, where we would be away from the elements and have plenty of space to work. The young bear's body showed no visible external signs of damage.

Gord provided details: "We've been carrying out trials on bear deterrents about half an hour east of here. We have been using those rubber bullets that were developed for crowd control and have been used in Northern Ireland."

The reason that this bear died had everything to do with the increasing incursion of people into polar bear habitat in the north and the need to keep bears and humans apart and safe without killing either one. Encounters were expected to increase, which was the reason that Gord's research was initiated. He was charged to find the most effective way to reduce human-bear encounters.

Part of the problem was that oil had been discovered in the region in the 1920s and '30s. Serious exploration of the region began in 1961, when it was discovered that most of the reserves lay offshore under the ice. In 1973 the world's first artificial island, made of thickened ice and strong enough to support a full-size oil rig, was built in the Beaufort Sea.

On January 5, 1975, 18-year-old Richard Pernitzky, who had been on an oil rig near Inuvik in the Northwest Territories, was killed by a polar bear when he was working on one of the outbuildings. A local trapper and his helpers tracked and eventually shot the bear while it was still carrying what remained of the young man's body. What a gruesome sight that must have been!

As reported in the *Vancouver Sun* on January 7 and 9 that year: "Three tags attached to the bear's ear showed that it had been tranquilized and removed from civilization at least three times."

It was obviously a recidivist bear similar to those I had dealt with in Jasper and Banff in 1976 and '77. It had been chased off only two days before the tragedy of Richard's death.

The reason this particular bear had not been "dealt with" was the law in place at the time that only an Aboriginal person could shoot a polar bear. Indeed when it was shot, as the paper reported, "The bear was later shot by a Native flown in by the RCMP." There were no guns at any rig at the time, but a positive outcome of the event was that a gun was kept at each camp to be used by a qualified marksman in case of an emergency.

Gord had brought along one of the huge rubber bullets (also known as baton rounds) for our inspection. It felt, weighed and looked like an elongated hockey puck made of hard rubber that I could in no way compress. It was as long as the width of a man's hand—10 centimetres (4 inches)—and 3.5 centimetres (1.5 inches) in diameter.

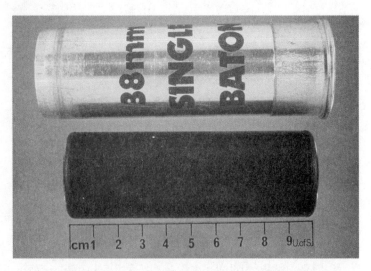

A baton round; not a nice thing to be hit with (10 cm = 4 in)

Gord explained, "These things were developed for crowd control. They are supposed to be fired into the pavement so as to ricochet up into an oncoming group of rioters. The muzzle velocity is slow enough that you can actually see them in flight, about one fifth the speed of a shotgun blast. They are very imprecise and inaccurate, but in the face of an onrushing crowd that isn't a consideration. In the last two years, we have used over 100 of them on the cape in a bear deterrent trial. They work well in moving a bear off a food source (a bait), and this is the first bear we have lost."

He went on to explain that the trial involved using a dead seal as bait, which was placed near a big metal cage. In the first trial, the researchers sat inside the cage (resembling shark cages that divers use), and the seal was placed about 30 metres (98 feet) away. As seals are the number one food item for bears, the design of the trial made perfect sense. The cage was used at first because the researchers didn't know if a polar bear would attack the shooter once it was hit with the rubber bullet. After testing the rubber bullet on about 50 bears with no ensuing charges from the bears, the researchers shot the bears with the rubber bullets from outside the test cage.

Gord went on, "My technician was handling the gun when this young bear turned up and began to sniff the seal. I was up in an observation tower above the test site recording reactions of the bears. They have an extraordinary sense of smell, said to be way more sensitive than a dog's, and he may have come a long way. Who knows? Anyway the technician pulled the trigger. The projectile is so slow that at the sound of the shot the bear lifted his head and turned slightly, which exposed his rib cage. As soon as the big bullet hit him just behind the elbow he ran off, but did not go far, only about 30 metres (98 feet). Then he stopped, shook himself and fell over dead."

It was time for me to start. No cuts were visible on the body indeed, even on close examination, I could see no signs of any external injury. But as I passed my hand over the bear's rib cage on the right hand side about halfway up, I could feel some movement of the bone over a small area, no more than about 5 centimetres (2 inches) across. It was just a slight crackle, more felt than heard.

The first step was to peel back the skin over his chest and belly. As I did, a large area of bruising over the chest where I had felt the crackling became obvious. Only the 6th rib was broken. Blood had spread from that spot.

An important feature was the lack of fat under the skin. In winter and spring, when the bears have been feasting on seals for a few months, the fat layer over the rump can be 10 centimetres (4 inches) thick, with a bit less farther forward. After summer on land and four months of fasting,

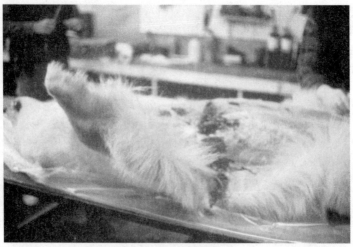

A big bruise under the skin over the 6th rib

the fat layer is greatly reduced or absent. If the fat had been present when this bear was shot, it might have acted as protective layer.

Inside the chest cavity I found almost 500 millilitres (2 cups) of blood and a small tear in the lung, as well as some bruising around it. Next I examined the heart, and I had never seen one that looked like it. The sac around the animal's heart, the pericardium, was swollen like a mis-shapen rugby ball and full of dark red fluid that was partly clotted blood. Inside was a single tear in the muscle of the heart, no more than 2 centimetres (.75 inches) long, but right through to the inner chamber.

It was not hard, although surprising, to figure out what had happened. The big bullet must have hit the chest end-on, right on the rib. Being so large and with no pointed end, the bullet stopped there and fell to the ground. The rest of the damage was caused by a shock wave that had not done any serious damage to thin-walled structures, especially the sac around the heart, but had ripped open the more solid muscle. The powerful pumping action of that muscle at once drove blood through the tear out into the sac. Although it is thin, the sac itself is tough, and only able to expand a little. Once it has reached its capacity to expand and the blood continues to be pumped into it, the pressure on the heart quickly prevents it from moving. This means that no blood can be pumped to the rest of the body, especially the brain. Death soon follows. The condition is called cardiac tamponade. I had never seen such damage before. We were intrigued and saddened by the results of the shooting.

Three weeks later, back in Saskatoon, I reported the case during Thursday morning rounds to my colleagues and the students at the vet college. This is standard practice in an academic environment, and the dean urged me to relate the event. I titled the little talk "Death of a Polar Bear: A Traumatic Event." It had been traumatic for the bear and soon afterwards for me. The room was packed. I'm not sure if that was because of the intended pun in the title or the mention of this charismatic species.

I have spoken to Gord a few times since our session over the post mortem table, images of which are seared into our memories. He told me that he used the bullets on at least 200 more bears in the early 1980s with no further deaths recorded. Gord has moved on without any censure from those events. He still studies bears, and is the lead grizzly bear scientist at the Foothills Research Institute in Alberta on secondment from the Alberta Government.

He wrote to me when I sent him an early draft of this chapter:

> There has been a lot of work done on the development and use of different types of bear deterrent systems since the early 1980s, and they are widely used in management jurisdictions today. However, without the early work on the effectiveness of these types of non-lethal deterrent systems, it is likely many more bears would have been killed [by rifle shots] rather than chased away.

That is the key point. If bears can be effectively deterred, they need not be killed. They are known to be highly intelligent, as anyone who has lived in the north will tell you. So a shot with a rubber bullet would likely only be needed once, at most twice, to teach the bears avoid contact with humans.

Like everything else, deterrent technology has come a long way since 1983. One reason is that the big gun used by Gord's technician is a restricted weapon and can only be used by a peace officer. Another is the advance in bullet type. A 12-gauge shell projectile composed of PVC plastic weighing only 403 grams (10.6 ounces) has been developed and works well.

Since 1983, no bullets of either kind have been used in Ireland; however, they are still in use elsewhere. Examples of the use of the plastic type include crowd control at the University of Nairobi in 1990, Quebec in 2001 and Hong Kong in 2014. Before the advent of rubber or plastic bullets, broom handles were used for riot control in Singapore in the 1880s. That sounds really scary.

When I followed up to get more background on the use of these huge projectiles, I found out more than I expected. During the "Troubles" (the conflicts in Northern Ireland between 1970 and 1989) when these bullets and the slightly smaller and slower plastic ones that replaced them were used, 17 people, eight of them children, died after direct hits. Dozens more were badly injured. Between 1970 and 1981, more than 98,000 of these bullets were fired. Seventeen deaths out of that many shots, one in nearly 6000, is statistically minute at just over 0.1 percent, but the statistics are irrelevant for the devastated families of those victims. As the saying goes, "The statistics may not be significant, but when it's you, it's 100 percent."

Ian Stirling, in his 1988 book *Polar Bears*, full of beautiful photos by Dan Guravich, tells how all but one of 404 bears hit with a rubber bullet fled immediately. He wrote that the exception was a large, thin adult male that did not move after five hits. Stirling did not mention the fatality I had worked, which would have counted as a second death.

He also describes all the other methods that Gord tried during his time at Cape Churchill. They included systems for detection of bears, not just polar bears, and deterrents. There were microwave detection units, trip wires, an electrified barbed wire fence, various noise-making devices including barking dogs and a set of floodlights. While the microwave and trip-wire systems were 100 percent effective in detection, the electrified fence was almost useless perhaps because it did not ground properly on the ice. Only the combination of the loud noise of the riot gun and the impact of the rubber bullets was routinely effective in 403 of the 404 bears hit. As Stirling wrote, "So Gordon went out to our observation tower…and turned it into something resembling a combat zone."

These two bears were the only known wild creatures to die after being hit by a rubber bullet.

Vandals at the Zoo

Some cases, such as the bull elk and his encounter with the wire, are short-term fires promptly doused by quick action. Two others were the direct result of vandalism. They were not so easily doused and had unhappy endings.

The first vandal was someone with both greed and a nasty turn of mind. The blue fox pen was raided. This beautiful cub had been born the previous spring to a red fox pair. When Sharon, who was on small animal duty, arrived in the morning she was met with the bloodied carcass near the gate. He had been skinned. It was a grizzly sight for all of us.

The director set up an altered shift rotation within a few minutes of our arrival at the coffee room. The keepers' hours were altered so that someone was on duty at night.

The second vandalism event, discovered a few nights later, was not caused by humans.

On the night Perry was on duty, he found during his rounds that two dogs had somehow got into the orphan deer shelter. Carnage had ensued. It was 8:00 in the evening. Perry immediately called Gerhard, who was working with him on the hoofstock section, and then called me. The scene at the shed was a nasty mess. Two orphaned white-tailed deer lay dead, one with its throat torn out and the other partially disembowelled. Three others were alive but torn up. One of them was past saving and died as I examined the other two.

The three of us took the little survivors to the office-cum-minor-surgery room. A sedative and pain killer helped them settle. We cleaned and stitched them up and injected an antibiotic. Both recovered, but we never found the dogs.

CHAPTER 25

Bison Studies
in Winter

My trips north to help in the study of wild bison occurred because Dr. Stacy Tessaro, right after his graduation from the Western College of Veterinary Medicine, went straight to a PhD course to study diseases that affect wild bison populations. His fieldwork took place in Wood Buffalo National Park, which straddles the border between Alberta and the Northwest Territories. Stacy met with Dr. Cormack Gates, the NWT biologist based in Fort Smith, a short distance east of the park just north of the boundary. He mentioned to Dr. Gates that a colleague had experience with wildlife immobilization and might be a good contact as the project expanded.

The diseases in question were tuberculosis and brucellosis. TB is well known, but brucellosis less so. It causes arthritis and has other nasty effects in most animals, including humans. In animals, the disease is most often transmitted through milk and grazing pastures contaminated by fluids that fall to the ground during the birthing process.

Transmission to humans occurs mostly through unpasteurized milk consumption. Sadly, the Haigh family had a close personal connection to the disease. My Aunt Joan had three mid-term miscarriages and bore a little girl, Phillipa, who survived only one day. All the deaths were the result of brucellosis because for many years, Joan drank unpasteurized milk straight from the farm. Happily two of her children, my cousins, were not affected.

Veterinarians are particularly at risk when exposed to birth fluids while assisting a cow to calve in countries where the disease is still endemic in cattle.

Following the well-documented wholesale slaughter of millions of bison in the 19th century, only an estimated 93 animals remained. Some were cared for on farms and ranches by well-meaning conservationists. Many of the calves were fostered on beef cows or suckled by dairy cows (in most instances there would have been no alternative). Between 1907 and 1909, 672 of those animals and their descendants were gathered together and shipped to Buffalo National Park near Wainwright, Alberta. The move occurred before tuberculosis and brucellosis had been eliminated from cattle herds by testing, culling and vaccination. It is almost certain that some of the cattle in those operations would have been infected. Inevitably some of the translocated bison acquired either or both infections from their bovine herd mates and brought the diseases to the park. They in turn spread the infections to others.

Some bison on those cattle ranches had almost certainly interbred with cattle. This led to contamination of the pure bison strain with cattle genes, explaining the finding of cattle genes in some bison herds.

In 1925 the government of Canada made a decision that Wes Olson, author, artist and dedicated long-time bison student, describes as "one of the worst decisions in the history of Canadian wildlife management." Between 1925 and 1928 the powers that be arranged for the translocation of 6673 plains bison from Wainwright north to the similarly but confusingly named Wood Buffalo National Park, where another sub-species, the wood bison, had long been resident. As Olson put it, "by the late 1930s the last [pure] wood bison was thought to have been lost due to hybridization with the introduced plains bison." As a result the wood bison sub-species was not only almost lost but infected with both diseases. The issue continues to be a problem in the new millennium.

In 1958 a remote herd of bison was located in the Needle Lake-Nyarling River region of Wood Buffalo National Park by Nick Novakowski of the Canadian Wildlife Service. Because of their geographic isolation, along with their physical traits, they were assumed to be pure wood bison.

Some of these individuals were captured. One group was moved across the Mackenzie River, which flows north and drains into the Arctic Ocean. Their destination was north and west of Great Slave Lake to the area now known as the Mackenzie Bison Sanctuary. Two groups went south, one to Elk Island National Park, where they thrive today, and another to the Moose Jaw Wild Animal Park in southern Saskatchewan. Those animals and their descendant groups that have subsequently been moved to other locations, such as the Toronto Zoo, are considered to be purebred wood bison.

Southern Saskatchewan has another, much darker, link to bison history. The province's capital city of Regina was originally known as "Pile of Bones" because of the huge masses of bison bones stacked nearby. "Pile of Bones" is the English translation of the Cree place name *oskana kâ-asastêki* that specifically refers to bison bones. The mounds were made when greed and cultural genocide perpetrated by European colonialists destroyed all but a few remnants of the once huge herds that followed the seasonal grazing. The bones were eventually used in the refining of sugar and to make fine bone china and fertilizer.

The number of bones can hardly be imagined. One example among many tells a small part of the story. The quantities were reported by weight in pounds. The Santa Fe Railroad reported more than 32 million pounds in the three years from 1872 to 1874.

Biologists working with bison wanted to know more about the Mackenzie Bison Sanctuary herd. The key questions were: Were the animals inbred, and were they free

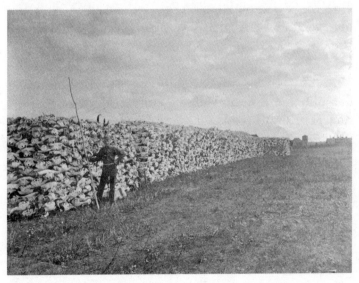

The 1890 photo by H.C.E. Lumsden of a pile of "buffalo" bones in Saskatoon

of the two diseases? The central part of the sanctuary is Falaise Lake, no more than 100 kilometres (60 miles) from the boundary of Wood Buffalo National Park. It is entirely possible that some infected plains bison from the park had migrated north and taken one or both scourges with them. Bison can swim with ease, and the river is frozen solid for most of the winter months, so such a migration is feasible. After all, migrations such as this and of much greater magnitude had occurred for centuries over most of North America.

Cormack called me soon after his conversation with Stacy to ask if I was available in late November or early December to work with his team. He explained that these months were the best period for the study. We also discussed drugs and equipment. I had found Carfentanil, the super-potent morphine-like drug that worked well for polar bear immobilization, to be an excellent choice for hoofed creatures. A small dose of cattle sedative also helped to smooth out the immobilization.

As for my equipment, the box containing the dart gun went into the hold on the flight north where no one could question it. The drugs had to go in my carry-on because if they froze in the hold, they would be useless.

Cormack, wearing a muskrat winter hat similar to those used by the Royal Canadian Mounted Police, met me at the small airport and took me to his home, where he began to tell me more about the project.

"As you know," he said, "my graduate student, Nick Larter, and I are currently studying the bison's diet and grazing habits. As part of that, we need collared animals so that we can trace where they go and how far they travel to find food at various times of year. I also want find out more about the disease situation in the sanctuary."

He dug out a large-scale map and showed me where we would be working.

"Where will we be based?" I asked. Cormack pointed to a spot on the map just across the river.

"We have a trailer at Fort Providence," he said. It was obvious that we had a long road trip ahead of us. The next morning we headed out on the lenghty drive north. Six hours later we reached the south shore of the frozen river.

There was a wide "lane" on the ice with lots of vehicle tracks between small spruce trees that had been cut off and "planted" on either side of the tracks. Some tracks were wide, likely made by large commercial freightliners bringing supplies to more northern communities, particularly Yellowknife. Others were made by smaller vehicles.

We turned left at the end of the crossing and were soon at the trailer. A helicopter was parked alongside. The next morning I loaded enough darts to have extra in case of a miss. Hopefully that would not happen. My target was pretty large.

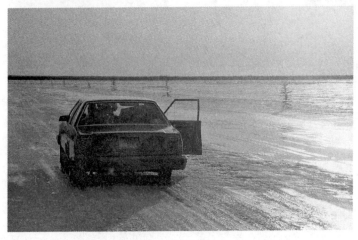

The ice bridge over the MacKenzie River showing trees used as markers

We headed west to the sanctuary. Ted Malewski, our pilot, and Cormack called out almost simultaneously, "There they are!"

From my position on the right rear seat no animals were visible, but a look over Ted's shoulder opened up the scene. Right in front of us was a herd of about 20 animals. I was surprised by how rapidly the huge beasts could move in the deep snow, but they were no match for the helicopter.

We selected a big bull at the rear of the group. It is much easier to hit the target when the machine is moving at the same speed as the animal. I fired as we gradually dropped to a safe distance above and to the left of him. A moment later we saw the dart sticking up from his backside.

We pulled away and up, so as to avoid stressing him unduly and watched as he ran off to join his group. Three minutes later he began to slow down and a minute later

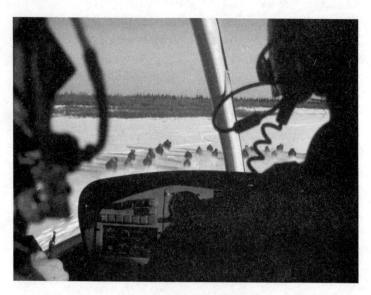

Bison on the run. The view over the pilot's shoulder.

stopped running then sank gently into the deep snow. Then it was a question of landing as close as possible, getting out of the chopper, and checking for safety before getting up to him.

First, I checked his breathing and pulse, then his temperature (not under his tongue or armpit). While the thermometer cooked, I went to his front end and collected a blood sample from his jugular vein. The sample would provide information about his disease status. The sample went into an inside pocket to prevent freezing.

Cormack and Nick placed a radio collar around his neck, tightened the nuts and bolts and inserted a red streamer into his ear. This technique was nothing new. Radio collars of the day enabled researchers to find an animal in a specific area. Once that is accomplished it is much easier to pick out the individual from a large herd if some

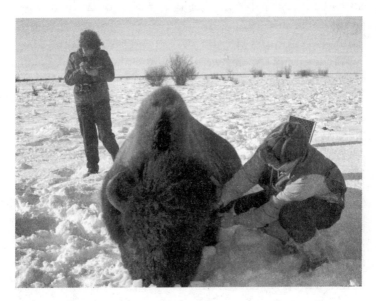

Bison health check

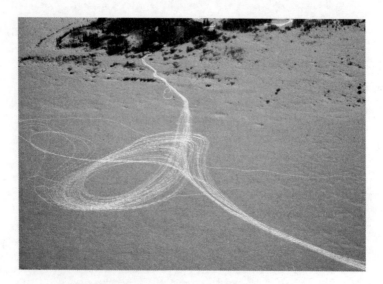

Bison tracks in the snow as they take evasive action

sort of highly visible marker is in place to catch the eye. With collar and ear tag in place, it was time for the antidote. Two minutes later he was up and heading out.

At the end of the day we took all the blood samples back to the trailer where we spun them in a centrifuge. We froze the serum from the samples, and I later took them to the vet college for analysis. We all hoped that they would be negative for disease. The results added to those collected by Stacy Tessaro were encouraging, but we needed more samples before we could be sure.

It was not always that simple to take down a single animal. Sometimes the small herds took evasive action, circling away from the noise and giant mosquito above them.

I was particularly interested to find out how the animals found enough food in the deep snow. Cormack was also interested, so we landed near a crater in the snow. He had a metre stick to measure the snow. It was 70 centimetres (27 inches) deep!

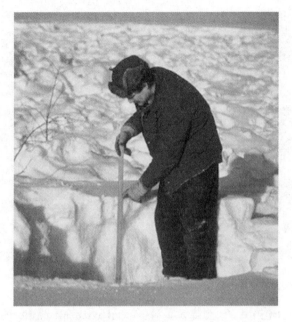

This bison-made crater is almost 1 metre (3 feet) deep.

Cormack explained: "They create the craters with sweeping movements of their huge heads. The result is that they can get down to the forage."

For one of my college student rotations, this one for wildlife, only one student signed up. Nigel Caulkett and I had first met when he was a stripling 14-year-old volunteer at the zoo. With clearance from the vet college Nigel was permitted to come north with me.

It was a bitterly cold month, and Nigel recalls, "I froze my ass off." He had never been that far north, but he was as keen as mustard and eager to learn. He recalled, when we chatted recently, that the rotation gave him "happy memories of a very exciting time in my life."

The capture process for females was much the same but with smaller doses of the drugs. Cormack also asked me to

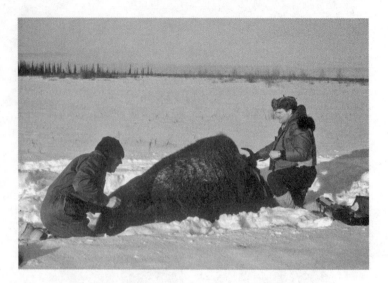

One hand warm to determine pregnancy

check for any pregnant cows. Even without the use of an ultrasound machine, diagnosing pregnancy is pretty simple. The best part of this process ensured that my left arm stayed warm.

We also captured and collared a few bison near Fort Liard, 500 kilometres (310 miles) west of Fort Providence. The backdrop of the mountains was the most striking difference between that spot and the Falaise Lake area.

We did have one disconcerting moment. After the antidote injection to a cow, we stepped back the regulation 20 or so metres (65 feet) and waited for her to get up. And waited…and waited. She should have risen after a minimum of five minutes, but after 10 minutes she was still down. I approached carefully and prodded her rear end. She turned her head to look, and I beat a hasty retreat. She struggled for a few more minutes, but she still couldn't stand. We waited a few minutes longer. We grunted and puffed as we tried to get her up on her chest. Still no luck.

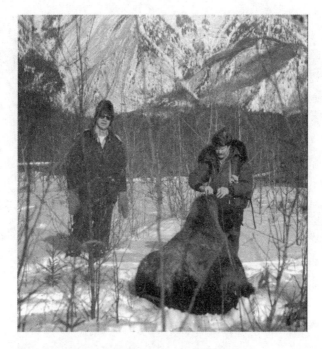

Backdrop of mountain scenery near Fort Liard

This was worrisome because we wondered if she had succumbed to the stress of capture.

Then the mental Rolodex kicked in. At vet school in Glasgow, now 20 years in the past, I had learned a way to help a recumbent dairy cow lying on its side to stand up. It was time for to use that know-how.

Ted pulled some heavy strapping from the compartment behind the backseat door, which we dragged over to the animal and slid under her neck and back to the level of her shoulders. We looped it around her lower foreleg and then pulled it over her upper shoulder. We stood well back, holding the end of the strap, and a hard pull rolled her up on to her brisket as the fulcrum of her shoulder provided the key point. Without a look back she jumped to her feet

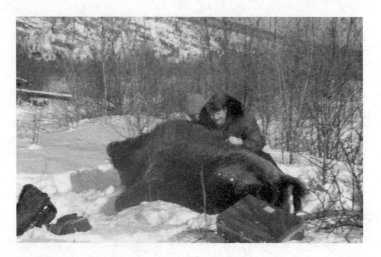

A failed attempt to get a cow to stand

and disappeared into the bush. Her collar continued sending its signal for many months.

Once Nick had finished his work, Petr Komers, a tall, blond Swiss scientist whose work in the sanctuary involved a study of the social role of bulls near Falaise Lake, began another study. He did much of his work during the summer months when we next got together.

Meanwhile it was back to Saskatoon for me. Little did I know what was in store.

Preventing a Rabies Outbreak

The very thought of rabies conjures horrific images of animals (and people) dying after a period of uncontrolled slobbering as wild seizures tear them apart. Once symptoms appear in any mammal, the disease is fatal. It kills at least 60,000 people worldwide every year but only a few in North America. Most cases are the result of dog bites, but in the prairies, most dogs are vaccinated. The striped skunk is one of the only carriers, but the disease can spread rapidly among skunk populations.

In the spring a skunk was seen climbing into the zoo over the perimeter fence. It was acting strangely so was shot within 10 minutes. The college soon confirmed the animal had rabies.

We decided that we needed to vaccinate of all the mammals in the collection, not urgently, because the unfortunate skunk didn't have time to make the rounds, but in case another showed up. I dared not use a vaccine that contained any form of live virus because nobody knew what effect, good or bad, it might have on the many species in the collection. Bad would mean an active infection caused by the live agent that might even spread through bites to other species. The decision came down to a killed version that would be safe under any circumstances. There was no information anywhere (pre-Google) on whether the vaccine would be effective as a preventative for zoo creatures, not even for wolves, dingoes and coyotes, all close relatives of the dogs for which the vaccine was designed. We would have to vaccinate everything twice, ideally at a 30-day interval to boost immunity. We also had to know if the animals already had any measurable level of protection before we started. Sounds simple, but it wasn't.

Some animals, particularly the carnivores, responded well to the vaccination. Their antibody levels increased markedly. A smaller proportion of the rest of the collection showed positive results but with a lower immunity. We had no idea if the vaccine was of any use for these animals, except that all staff felt a measure of comfort.

By the time we finished vaccinating all the animals, six months had gone by. By then I was back at the Mackenzie Bison Sanctuary for another 10-day stint.

CHAPTER 26

Summer Bison

In the interval between the rabies vaccination series, I joined Cormack at Fort Smith, and we headed out in his car to Fort Providence. By July the ice bridge across the Mackenzie River had melted, but the ferry solved the problem of getting across the water.

The Mackenzie Bison Sanctuary research was not finished. Petr needed more information about the study of reproductive behaviour. His main goal was to learn more about the bulls at the onset of the rut, which starts in late June and peaks in July and August. This meant that we needed to identify bulls earlier in the summer. At Providence we met up with Larry Penner, a skilled wildlife technician who had joined the team.

The capture procedure in summer was different. Rather than the helicopter, we used quad bikes and an Argo all-terrain vehicle to get to Falaise Lake. The Argo can traverse swampy areas—a considerable advantage around the edges of where the bison often like to feed.

The first thing I learned was that working in these conditions requires just as much protection as the winter gear needed in December. The protection involves lightweight clothing, long trousers tucked into good socks, a long-sleeved shirt and, most important by far, a hooded bug jacket soaked regularly in insect repellent. The mosquito is widely recognized as the "national bird" of the region, and black flies are fierce competitors for the title. It is said that if either or both of them could only cooperate, they could carry someone away never to be seen again. This delightful thought is reminiscent of New Zealand's Fiordland "where sandflies [go] about in mobs of thirty million and [eat] everything that the mosquitoes overlook...." It took me only a day to learn why the local NWT *Tabanids*, known as horseflies, are called bulldogs. Their bite feels as if a drill bit is being driven into the skin.

In this part of the study we approached the bison using whatever cover was available. The animals were immobilized from the ground using one of two kinds of darting equipment. For animals at ranges above 15 or 20 metres (50 or 65 feet) the dart gun was the same one used from the helicopter. If distances were longer, the range dial could be cranked up to 50 or 60 metres (165 or 200 feet).

At shorter distances, a modification of my blowgun came into play. With the barrel extended to 1.8 metres (6 feet), a shot out to 20 metres (65 feet) was possible. If the puff was hard enough and the pipe elevated at the front end, with practice the dart arced into the target. However, getting into close range led to two kinds of stress, not so much for the bison as for the team.

We often saw bulls lying well out in open areas, a long way from any bushy vegetation, usually wallowing in dry,

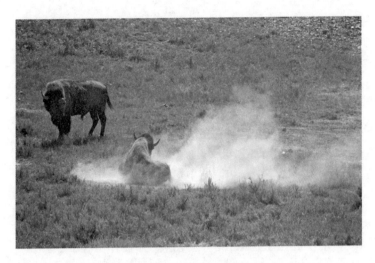

Nothing like a good sand bath (© Johane Janelle)

sandy areas. They were undoubtedly trying to protect themselves from those hordes of blood-sucking insects.

My suggestion to the crew, based on my experience of animal behaviour after 20 odd years of work with many species, was that I approach these bulls by walking slowly out in the open and get close enough to use the blowgun. We all knew that the fully mature bison had little to fear from predators. Nonetheless Cormack, Petr and Larry looked at me as if to ask, "Have you lost your mind?"

With blowgun in hand I set off out into the meadow from the bushes where the others were hiding. Sometimes the bulls were at least 200 metres (660 feet) from us. Larry loaded his rifle and assured me that if things went awry, he would take action.

The upright walk, slowly, very slowly out into the open, involved a route that started at the narrower end of an egg shape, with the other, rounded end (where the bison lay relaxing) as the destination. Viewed from above, the route is reminiscent of Jonathan Swift and his satirical view of politics and Gulliver's experiences with the divided community of the "Big-Ender" and the "Small-Ender" Lilliputians who could not decide which end of a soft-boiled egg should be cracked before being eaten. This was definitely a Big-Ender situation.

The bulls looked me over once but mostly ignored me. Once or twice a single animal, often in a group of six or seven, stood up and took a look, his tail at half-mast. He was curious. When this happened, I crouched, pulled up some grass and tossed it over my head. The hope with this seemingly daft action was to fool him and his buddies into thinking that some harmless creature was passing by. As they had almost certainly never seen a human, the idea worked.

I know that the most critical signal to look for lies at the rear end, not the head. When a bison is relaxed, his tail hangs almost straight down. If the tail is at half-mast, the bull is interested. Be careful! You are close enough. When the base of the tail is at the ten o'clock position, the bull is feeling tense, and it's time to get out of there. As for a lift to a vertical position, author and artist Wes Olson quotes Vern Ekstrom of Custer State Park in South Dakota who wrote: "There's only two reasons why a buffalo raises his tail. The first is to charge, and the second is to discharge." If the tail is in upright position, with the head lowered and back arched, and accompanied by what looks like a flag waving in the wind, trouble is brewing. I had no intention of being the object of such an attention. My 90-kilo (198-pound) frame would soon look like a strawberry mousse.

In every case, the inquisitive bull soon lay down, allowing the walk-cum-crawl to restart. Eventually, I could begin to close the oval shape of my approach and get within 20 metres (65 feet). Sometimes the bulls just looked

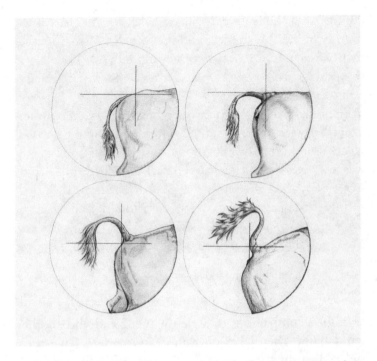

This illustration by artist Wes Olson shows the four tail positions that indicate a bison's state of mind.

me over and did not even bother to stand up. This was a nuisance. The target area was much reduced if the bull remained bedded down. I had to wait for at least one to stand again to get a clear broadside shot. As soon as this happened, the blowgun came up, followed by a hard puff, sending the dart on its way towards the heavy muscles of the hind end.

Most of the bulls took no notice, and none threatened me. Perhaps they thought the needle prick was just another bloody bulldog. As before, they soon started to stagger; some even left the sand bath and lay down. At this point the quad bikes left the shelter of the trees to join in the work. The noise and the strange machines persuaded

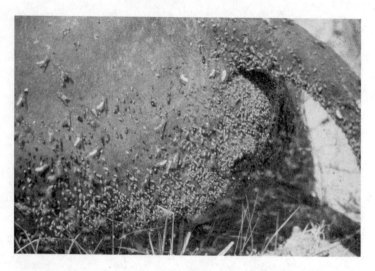

Black flies, mosquitoes and "bulldogs" on the rear of an immobilized bison

the bull's companions to leave the scene and find another sand bath. They were no doubt annoyed to have their siesta disturbed.

The first thing that happened in summer to an immobilized animal was the arrival of hundreds, maybe thousands, of airborne pests. They swirled around his whole body like a cloud. When he had settled and we could safely approach, the real extent of the invasion was obvious. He could no longer use his tail as a whisk. The invading army had landed.

One bull, lying with his companion near some bushes, led to an interesting encounter. I had darted him while he stood, then waited the standard five minutes for him to lie down. The two bulls had moved off into the brush. Cormack and I separated and went searching for my patient. Soon I came upon him lying under a tree and called out to Cormack.

A second later he called back, "Jerry, I've found him. The dart is still in his backside."

It was sheer luck that my undarted bull was facing away so that he didn't see me. I was well inside the fight zone, so a hasty but quiet retreat was in order. Had he seen the unwelcome intruder, the paperwork for Cormack would have been time-consuming and would have cut into the research program.

There was one extra thing that needed study. Only a small group had been translocated from the Nyarling River. Some inbreeding must have occurred, but did it have any serious effects?

The plan was two-fold. We could collect semen from the bulls during the latter part of the rut, in late August or early September, and evaluate the samples right away to see if they were normal. At the same time we'd measure the size of their scrotums and check to see if the animals had the normal number of its contents. The jargon for those that did not was "one stoner." No doubt this derived from the Allied soldiers' World War II song mocking Hitler and his cronies. In my relatively youthful days, 30 or more guys had sung the tune at many a post-rugby, beer-assisted evening:

> *Hitler has only got one ball,*
> *Göring has two, but they're too small,*
> *Himmler has something sim'lar,*
> *But poor old Goebbels has no balls at all.*

Only two bulls matched Hitler's alleged anatomical deficit.

Once the bull was down it became even more of a team effort than merely putting on a radio collar. Larry and

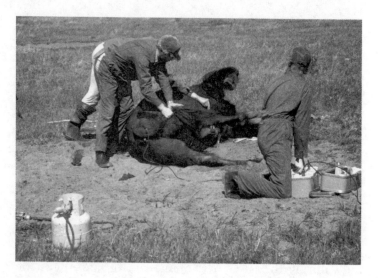

Semen collection at Falaise Lake

Cormack joined forces to hold the bull's hind leg out of the way.

The equipment used has two parts to it. The probe looks just like a 40-centimetre long, 8-centimetre (16- x 3-inch) diameter bomb with three embedded metal rods on one side. These days such an object would not be easy to load onto an aircraft because security is so much tighter. The electrical box has several dials and a meter that reads out the current being used. If both pieces were loaded together at an airport, it's certain that two grim-looking individuals would be asking some serious questions off in a side room. One might find oneself incarcerated for a time and unable to board. I like to imagine the effects of a demonstration with a security person holding the probe. Surprise? A smile? Probably not. Outrage? Maybe fury?

To use the equipment, the lubricated probe is inserted into the rectum (metal rods down to stimulate the interior nerves and organs that lead to erection) and the current is gradually increased at each turn until the desired results are achieved. The semen is then collected in a test tube. We soon had our sample and had measured the scrotum. Only two of the 15 bulls tested were one-stoners, and all but one of the semen samples were normal.

Cormack wanted to continue the summer work the following year, and because I was away in Africa on a sabbatical he invited Nigel, who was now fully qualified. The team was able to collect semen from another 11 bulls. The results of the tests were similar to the first ones.

Nigel recalls, with deadpan humour, how security opened his bags at check-in. Twelve other passengers were standing in line behind him. "I had to explain, in front of everyone, that one puts the probe up the bull's butt, hooks up the orange box and electrocutes the bull until he ejaculates. I did eventually board, but the flight was a tad delayed."

The results of the disease tests collected by the team, from more than 150 bison in five years, showed that all were free of both tuberculosis and brucellosis. At this point government authorities, in consultation with Cormack, made a decision intended to keep the sanctuary animals disease free: if any bison is seen wandering between the park and the sanctuary, in either direction, it is shot. Since that time, the herd has increased in size and now a highly controlled and limited hunting season has been opened.

My last opportunity to work with Cormack and wood bison in the NWT occurred at the end of the summer of 1989, the year that the Moose Jaw Wild Animal Park closed for good. The park, owned by the Saskatchewan provincial government, was one of the three destinations to which the wood bison were shipped after the remnant population near the Nyarling River had been discovered in the late 1950s. The government made the wise decision to send them back north rather than sell them or move them to another zoo where they might easily hybridize with plains bison.

After appropriate testing, the remaining dozen head were trucked more than 2500 kilometres (1500 miles) to Nahanni Butte, some 500 kilometres (300 miles) west of Fort Providence. There had been an earlier translocation (in 1980) of 28 animals from Elk Island National Park to the area. The Moose Jaw animals were released into a 0.4-hectare (1-acre) pen in a so-called "gentle" release. This ensured that they would not scatter to the four winds.

The gentle release involved feeding the animals hay until they had settled, at which time the gate was opened and feeding continued until green forage was available.

Another group of 59 animals was released north of Fort Liard, some 100 kilometres (60 miles) south of Nahanni nine years later. It is not known if the two groups linked up, but in 2011, the total population was estimated to be

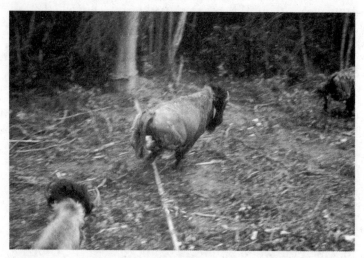

Wood bison release at Nahanni in 1989

400 animals. That same year, in the Nahanni area, a hunting quota of 11 head was set.

Like me, Cormack has retired and has been able to indulge in his passion for fly-fishing. Nigel has gone on to a spectacular career in many countries, concentrating on the development of more effective and safer drug combinations for wildlife capture. He has told me that his work stems from that first trip to the North. He has dealt with the cold by purchasing better clothing (better than most students can afford) and has worked "Way up north, north to Alaska" as the classic song goes, and in Canada's High Arctic.

In his research, Petr found that the old bulls in the bison sanctuary were the real breeders; they were the better fighters and won the mating rights. However, when Petr controlled the bull age composition in an experimental captive population, he found that when young bulls had the opportunity to mate, they did the service but did not do so in as orderly a fashion as the old bulls in the wild. These youngsters, perhaps equivalent to human teenagers, ran around more frantically and created commotion, sometimes dangerous to the females, resulting in greater risks and energy exertion for the cows.

Petr is now based in Calgary and works as a scientific advisor to review boards, municipalities and local communities.

A Puzzle Helped by
Laboratory Work

Another fire began with a single case. It started as a slow-burner, smouldered, became serious and was extinguished with a treatment developed for humans.

An elk calf arrived at the zoo, brought to us by an officer of the Provincial Department of Natural Resources. He explained that it had been found near a dead female that had been hit by a vehicle. No one had any idea how long the calf had been without milk.

The little calf could not have been more than a week old. After some initial reluctance it soon attached itself to the rubber nipple at the end of a bottle of milk replacer. We'd had more experience than we wanted in the raising of deer, particularly orphan white-tailed deer fawns, to be fazed by the standoffishness of this calf. The only difference was the size of the orphan.

Every year, well-meaning but sadly mistaken members of the public brought fawns to the zoo. They would usually say something like, "We found the poor little thing in the grass and there was no mum around, so we thought we had better rescue him." The mistake was not knowing that deer fawns fit into the category of so-called "hiders." After a fawn has nursed, the doe leaves it to hide until its next appointment. However, sometimes the arrival of a fawn, or occasionally fawns, made more sense. Spring is seeding time, and if farmers out in their big tractors saw a dappled youngster lying in front of the machine they would good-heartedly pick it up and bring it to us.

Our new arrival soon caught on to the idea that a keeper with a bottle in hand was good news, and it more-or-less vacuumed the milk, seeming not to realize when its ration was finished. After a few fruitless sucks it then stood still. This gave the keeper a chance to apply a damp cloth to its rear end, thus both cleaning it and stimulating it to empty its bowels.

For a week, all seemed well; the little elk was frolicking and interacting with the fawns that were housed in the same enclosure. One morning 10 days after she arrived, she ran up as usual to her bottle, took a few sucks and quit. That afternoon she did exactly the same thing. In the morning Gerhard found her lying dead.

By mid-afternoon I knew what had killed her. Standing in the post mortem room at the vet college, suitably dressed in coveralls and rubber boots, I watched as pathologist Garry Wobeser, who specialized in wildlife cases, opened her up. Even with my limited pathology education it was easy to see what had happened. A large ulcer had eroded through her stomach wall, and she had died from a combination of loss of blood and shock due to the acid fluids of her stomach entering her abdomen.

Not long afterward, one of the two orphan fawns at the zoo developed the same symptoms, taking a few sucks at the bottle and then backing off. The fawn's discomfort was plain to see. It kept getting up and down, kicking at its belly and even looking round at its side. The heart and lungs sounded normal, and the thermometer stewed long enough to give an accurate reading. But the penny dropped when I extracted the thermometer and smelled the repulsive odour of the feces on the glass. It is a smell that vets know only too well. Not only did it stink but it was black instead of the creamy brown of a calf on a milk diet. Such an odour may have other causes, but the foul smell is usually associated with bleeding high up in the intestinal tract, often from damage to either the stomach or the duodenum.

Deer and other ruminants do not have a "stomach" in the human sense, but the so-called fourth stomach, the abomasum, performs the same function. It secretes chemicals, most notably acid, that help digestion. When the youngster is still drinking milk, the first three stomachs have no function. They are bypassed as the milk goes directly to the abomasum.

Stress leading to stomach inflammation (gastritis) or, less commonly, ulcers can be a cause of the signs shown by the little patient. Being orphaned and then offered unnatural milk by a human can surely be classed as double whammy.

There are other causes of the foul-smelling feces. Cancer is a consideration but could hardly apply in one so young. Bacteria may also cause an intestinal ulcer. The most famous demonstration of a bacterium called *Helicobacter pylori* occurred when Australian scientist Dr. Barry Marshall drank a beaker full of this culture. He became ill a few days later, and he identified large numbers of the bacterium in his own stomach. He then self-medicated with an antibiotic and recovered. That brave experiment eventually led to a cure for humans.

However, the link between *H. pylori* and stomach trouble had not been accepted in the medical community of the day and had certainly not appeared in the veterinary literature. The best treatment in humans was a drug commercially known as Tagamet that reduced the amount of acid in the stomach. I knew about the product, whose chemical name is cimetidine, and decided that it might be worth a try on the little deer.

Faye Kernan, the pharmacist at the vet college, was able to obtain some Tagamet from the suppliers. It came only in little vials for injection, designed for a single human dose. The weight of an average western human in the early 1980s was considered to be 70 kilograms (155 pounds) (it is now more than 80 [175]). Our deer fawns, only a few days old, weighed less than 5 kilograms (10 pounds). We then had to guestimate the dosage: 70 divided by 5 equals 14. It is impossible to take 1/14 of the volume of one cc with any accuracy using a syringe. I opted for 1/10 and gave each of the four orphans in the pen an injection. We repeated the injections in the afternoon. The results were not far short of miraculous. The next morning the reluctant fawn came quickly up to the keeper when he called. It enthusiastically emptied the entire bottle in one uninterrupted guzzle. Based on more guesswork and the package information from the drug company, I continued the daily treatment for 10 more days. Along with the cimetidine, it seemed wise to start a regime of antibiotics for the youngster.

Three days into the process, Faye said to me, "Jerry, did you know that we can get a generic form of cimetidine that comes as tablets? It is much cheaper than the injections. I can easily get some from one of the pharmacies in town."

The tablets arrived the next day. The human dose is one tablet taken once or twice a day, meaning that each pill had to be divided into 10 equal parts. The task proved impossible; each cut with a scalpel caused a few tiny crumbs of drug to fall away. Ten roughly equal sections would have to do. The keepers then crushed each tiny portion between two teaspoons and tipped it into the morning bottle of milk. This technique can justly be called crude, but the fawn recovered fully.

Over the next two summers we were able to use our experience in eight other young ruminants, all under three months of age—another fawn, three moose calves and three elk. We also applied it to two muskoxen that were part of a herd being studied by my colleague Peter Flood and his graduate student Jan Rowell.

At the annual meeting of zoo veterinarians, held that year in Seattle, I mentioned these cases to a few vets who specialized in marine mammal work. They told me that stomach and duodenal ulcers are seen in almost 75 percent of rescued sea lions on the west coast of the U.S. Cimetidine proved effective in several cases.

CHAPTER 27

Bison in Art

One of the earliest paintings Jo and I purchased in Canada was an evocative winter scene of bison crossing a frozen lake. The work, by Conrad Mieschke, titled "Northern Spirits," caught our imaginations, and we have been fascinated by bison ever since.

Imagine yourself as a weekend caver, a speleologist or spelunker. It is the year 1994. You are in the Ardèche region of southern France following an air current that comes from between a rubble of stones at the end of a small cave in a limestone cliff above the Ardèche River. You are Eliette Brunel, a member of the three-person team led by Jean-Marie Chauvet. Your colleague, Christian Hillaire, is the third member of the group.

After unblocking the passage, crawling through it and climbing down into a cave below with a spelunking ladder, you see a mass of crystal deposits and signs of previous human visitors in the form of cave paintings.

You cannot contain your excitement and shout out to your companions.

This is precisely what happened to the small team, and it was only the beginning of an amazing journey through time. Time that stretches back 36,000 years and shows astonishing cave art that is not only the oldest known to archeologists but arguably some of the most accomplished ever seen.

As Joshua Hammer tells it in his *Smithsonian Magazine* article, Jean Clottes, the world-famous pre-historian was dragged away from his family's New Year's gathering to help with examination of the brand new complex. He, too, had to wriggle his way through the passage, crawling to enter the cave.

Soon afterwards and before the find was made public, a steel door was put in place to prevent public access. This was done to preserve the art from the drastic changes that such an opening would bring. The climate of a cave is mostly stable and has remained so for millennia. Numerous visitors would have added to the changes in temperature and humidity as happened to the famous Lascaux cave that eventually had to be closed off, even though most of its splendid art has been preserved. The Chauvet Cave is now officially named Grotte Chauvet-Pont d'Arc. Le Pont d'Arc is the stunning natural arch bridge in the valley next to the cave, and Chauvet because the leader of the three discoverers was Jean-Marie Chauvet. The cave has never been open to the public and will not be.

The most famous art in the cave is the set on the so-called horse panel. There are also many lion and cave bear pictures; a few aurochs, the extinct cattle-type creature that is thought to be the ancestor of today's domestic cattle; and some rhino, a few with horns so long that they are either the artist's fancy or an ancient version of an animal that has lasted, in varying forms, throughout the ages.

For the African in me, the most fascinating rhino picture shows two animals, nose-to-nose and horn-to-horn. Drawn in that ancient era, they are almost certainly woolly rhinoceros, ancestors of today's species. Given what I have witnessed and what is generally known about rhino behaviour today, and assuming that its belligerent nature is one feature inherited from its ancestors, there is little doubt that they are fighting. The "fight" may even be a part of the vigorous foreplay that occurs when today's African species feel randy.

Some of the 425 pictures have been carbon-dated at something more than 35,000 years. Other much "younger" pictures were drawn 5000 years later.

In order to bring the story to the public while preserving the art, filmmaker Werner Herzog decided to make a documentary about the find. French authorities gave him permission to film in the cave in 2011 under rigorous conservation conditions.

Clottes also photographed the entire array of paintings. On finding Clottes photos online, it took me only the briefest of moments to recognize that many of the cave's art works were created by talented artists who were also keen observers of animal life. Several drawings look like modern bison. Because of their age and location in France, they might be the related steppe wisent, but they look very much like the bison we know in North America. The difference between one of the Chauvet bison and the other bison images in the cave is that the animal has more than four legs possibly to show it was walking or running. Some are dark, as if in the foreground. Others are pale and not filled in. The same technique was also applied to a reindeer in the End Chamber.

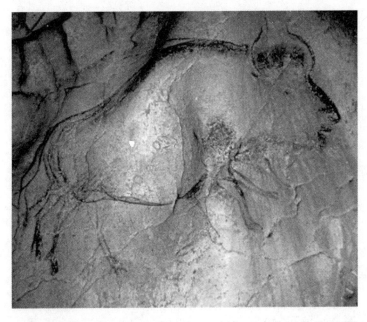

A Jean Clottes photo of a depiction of a running bison in the Chauvet Cave in France

In an expensive but brilliantly conceived move, the French government has spent almost €55 million ($62.5 million USD) on the creation of a fully realized copy of the cave. Located only 5 kilometres (3 miles) from the original site, it has been in the works for eight years and was opened to the public early in 2015. A team of 500 people—architects, artists, engineers and special effects experts—collaborated in the endeavour. To ensure that the replica matches the original, laser-scanning techniques were used. Experts were allowed into the real cave in short bursts of no more than two hours at a time to do the scans, which took some 700 hours to complete. Jean Clottes, in his capacity as a preeminent cave expert in France was a leading team member as president of the scientific committee for the replica.

~

Now imagine yourself as a six-year-old all those years ago. You and your daredevil young friends creep through the trees and bushes following the clan shaman Suviyan at a safe distance to see where she goes every day. She disappears down a cliff into the rocks at a cave entrance. A week later, at dusk on midsummer's night she leads her clan into that secret place where none dare enter alone for fear of demons.

She holds a magical cave bear bone bound with sticks that she dips into the fat of a fierce lion that your father killed in the cold weather. With a spark from a flint stone, she sets it alight at the cave entrance. She guides everyone though the dark tunnel as the flames light up the walls and ceiling.

You walk between your mum and dad, holding their hands. You remember your last visit a year ago, when Suviyan showed you her picture of two huge rhinos fighting. You remember hearing their grunts and squeals as they faced one another, horns clashing. Then the heavy sounds of the fight. You were frightened, but you somehow forgot to mention this terror to any of your friends.

What will you see this year?

Suddenly the sound of a charging animal comes down the length of the cave.

The light from the shaman's flare moves across another lion's head. She steps forward and waves it in front of a huge bison that is running just in front of you.

Have you shut your eyes and turned your face into dad's deer-hide coat?

~

Fast forward. Archaeologists tell us that the bison reached North America by crossing the Bering Land Bridge some 10,000 years ago. In the intervening 25,000 years, the steppe wisent drawn in what has become France has had time to both evolve into the creature we now know as bison and to do so over 8500 kilometres (5000 miles). That is a long, slow walk.

The account matches nicely with the Tsuu T'ina Nation (formerly Sarcee) story of how the buffalo reached the area south and west of today's Calgary. In 1995 Grant MacEwan, in his book *Buffalo Sacred and Sacrificed* tells how 84-year-old David One Spot related the legend of that arrival to the Calgary Rotary Club in 1956.

> *The buffalo came from a far land and it was like this. There were two brothers, who, like some white boys, didn't get along very well. The older boy said to the younger one "You climb that tree and see what is in the eagle's nest." The younger one did what he was told to do and climbed but the older one immediately cut the tree down, and both the tree and boy fell in the river. Clinging to the tree the younger brother floated far away to a strange land where he thought he was dying from starvation.*
>
> *By good fortune, the boy was discovered by a beautiful girl who thought he was dead. But on the chance that there was still some life in the body, she took it to her home and administered life-giving steam baths. The treatment proved miraculous and the boy recovered. Then, of course, he married the girl.*
>
> *In this far-off land, the boy was to see animals that were new to him, among them the buffalo which the people rode whenever*

they wished to travel. But in time the young man became lonely for his own country and persuaded his wife to return there with him. Riding two buffalo, they followed the river all summer and finally came to the part he recognized as his own. But sad news awaited him. The game animals had almost disappeared and the people were starving. To try and take his people back to the part where the buffalo abounded was not likely to succeed. It would be too far. But on a still night when the moon was full, the young man's wife went to the top of the highest hill, faced her land of her birth and called, "Buffalo! Buffalo! Buffalo!"

The next day herds of buffalo thundered in from the east. Hungry people ate buffalo meat, something they had never tasted before, and the herds that had answered the young wife's call remained to live thereafter in the country of plains and foothills. That's how the buffalo happened to be in the these parts where the white man first saw them.

–Old David One Spot of the Sarcees said so.

~

Fast-forward another 10,000 years (give or take 92).

We find a charming letter in our mailbox. It is signed Clarence Tillenius. He writes in a sprawling but legible hand soon after my first book, *Wrestling With Rhinos*, has been published. He not only writes but pastes photocopied snippets from the book among the sentences. We arrange a visit with him at his home in Winnipeg.

At 92 years of age he is working on a panel of bison pictures. It is a 150-centimetre long by 30-centimetre (60- x 12- inch) tall panorama depicting scenes of the animals in various situations. For me, the most memorable is of a warrior armed with a long gun as he rides down a running bison. As we chat he puts some finishing touches to the fine black hairs on the animal's mane. Jo asks how he is going to use the piece.

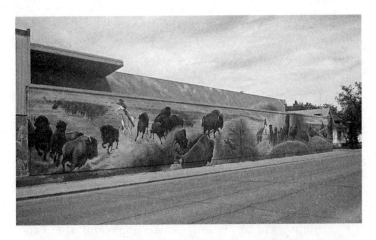

Charlie Johnston's mural at 1881 Portage Avenue in Winnipeg from the work of Clarence Tillenius

"Oh, a young fellow is going to project it onto a supermarket wall. He will do it on a moonless night from across the street. It will be huge, and then he will paint the wall using the projected image as the foundation," he says.

Given his age we wonder what he meant by a young fellow. Maybe anywhere from 20 to 60?

The supermarket stands at 1881 Portage Avenue. Anyone driving on Canada's cross-country Number One highway through the city could stop and marvel at the work. The huge painting might even cause traffic jams. The artist who transferred Clarence's work, with minor changes to fit the scene, is Charlie Johnston. As Johnston wrote:

> *Clarence is a naturalist as much as he is a painter or artist.... If the bison were in a stampede, all of the other animals scatter. Here, it's the fox and the hare; and they had to be in synch with that, moving away from the stampede. If wolves were squaring off against bison, it had to be a bison that had been separated from the herd. The composition of the design had to make sense naturalistically to Clarence.*

We learned several things from Clarence. He had worked across Canada from coast to coast. He lost his right arm in a logging accident before World War II, and he dealt with that impediment by teaching himself to paint left-handed.

Much later, and none of it from the man himself, we learned several other things about his artistic life. He created 200 large oils of Canadian wildlife across Canada. He was honoured by a variety of organizations, and these culminated in his being awarded the Order Of Canada in 2006, the year we met him.

After we admired the work he was doing and had taken him for lunch at the Pavilion Gallery in Assiniboine Park, we went upstairs where he showed us more of his paintings. A small representation of his work occupies the entire second floor of the gallery. There we saw the originals of many of the magazine covers he did for *Country Guide* and *The Beaver* over a 40-year span.

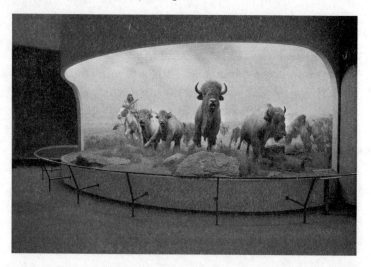

Tillenius's bison diorama in the Manitoba Museum. Reproduced with permission of the Manitoba Museum.

Clarence asked if we had time to visit the Manitoba Museum where, as he put it, he had a few things on display. As we entered, the receptionist smiled and greeted him as a friend. His "few things" were a series of wildlife dioramas. Two stood out for me. In his design and execution of two moose at the edge of a water body, I could hardly make out the border between the taxidermy work of the animals, the bulrushes, the sedge grasses and the actual painted background.

His work on a herd of bison being run down by a gun-toting hunter on a horse is extraordinary. It is no wonder his dioramas were declared National Treasures by the Canadian Museum of Nature in Ottawa.

Unfortunately, the gallery had no bison pictures for sale at a price we could afford. We did, however, purchase two others. The oil was a scene of pronghorn antelope in the

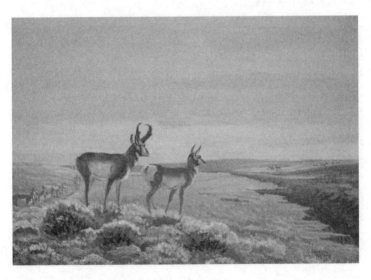

Pronghorn on the alert. Perhaps overlooking the Frenchman Valley in Southern Saskatchewan. Courtesy of the estate of Clarence Tillenius.

southern prairies, the other a field pencil sketch of a polar bear and her cubs.

Tall mustachioed Wes Olson, seldom seen without a Stetson on his head, and his photographer wife Johane Janelle were friends with Tillenius. This comes as no surprise since Wes has spent much of his life studying and drawing bison.

Only an unlikely confluence of the planets can explain how three people who both own work by and are enthusiastic about Clarence would end up at the same banquet table for eight at the 2015 bison conference in Saskatoon with more than 200 attendees. Conrad Schiebel was the third guest. His father-in-law supported Tillenius, and his

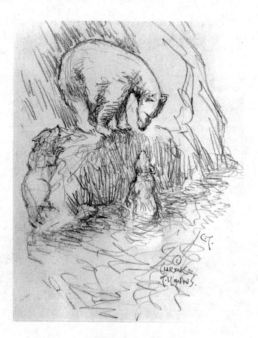

A polar bear and her cubs. Courtesy the estate of Clarence Tillenius.

family have the great good fortune to own some of the artist's work.

As we chatted of things bison and Tillenius, Conrad asked Wes about his history and particularly how long he had been drawing and painting.

"Probably since age six," he replied.

Wes started his working life as a wildlife researcher and became a park warden. He recounts with humour how he first met Clarence: "I was working in Elk Island National Park and checking back trails on my quad. I came around a corner and found an illegally parked RV. I was all set to charge the driver when I saw that he was working at an easel and painting a herd of bison. We chatted for quite some time."

When asked if he had charged the famous artist for illegally being in a restricted area of the park he replied, with

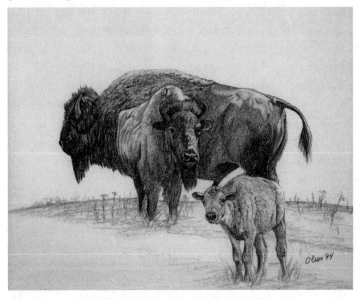

Wes Olson's drawing of three bison on pasture

a smile and a shake of his head, "No. We just chatted about this magnificent creature." Wes retired from the park service in 2012, so he can tell this story without fear of reprisal for failure of duty.

Wes and Johane now live in the tiny Saskatchewan village of Val Marie near the U.S. border. This puts them alongside one of the newest National Parks in Canada, the Grasslands National Park, through which runs the Frenchman River. It comes as no surprise that the park is now home to a herd of bison. Wes had a critical role in the translocation of this group of animals from his former stomping grounds in Elk Island.

The couple has collaborated in the publication of a book that is an essential guide to bison society. The beautiful work is full of Wes' art and Johane's photographs. Clarence Tillenius wrote the foreword that not only describes Olson's addiction to bison but also describes his fascination and work with many other wild creatures.

Olson and Janelle's book has many of Wes' gorgeous graphite pencil drawings and their photos that match the "Northern Spirit" feel of Conrad Mieschke's painting. In Wes' writing, the book gives a tidy summary about the bison's role in history, its behaviour and biology and particularly the need for people to understand its behaviour relative to human safety.

~

From the earliest times, bison have roamed across an enormous swatch of North America. Then came greed and both direct, via sanctioned murder, and indirect, through the wholesale slaughter of animals, cultural genocide by European invaders. There are many publications that describe the killing of thousands of the hardy creatures that were the main source of food, shelter and clothing of the Native people.

Two such books tell that story in different ways. Their creators are artists in a different genre, but nonetheless artists—Grant MacEwan and Peter Erasmus. They were respectively a writer and a storyteller.

The first thing one sees on opening MacEwan's book *Buffalo Sacred and Sacrificed* before even reading the chapter headings, are two of Wes Oslon's pictures. MacEwan has pulled together many stories of the history and near-ultimate demise of the buffalo. Of the many accounts over and above David One Spot's story, excerpted earlier, struck me as an example of how much the First Nations People hunted and used the animals.

In his chapter titled "The Big Buffalo Hunt—Red River Style," MacEwan recounts how, in 1840, 400 mounted hunters produced 1375 tongues, the delicacy part of the carcass, by evening. It must have been a mad chase. He tells, in another chapter, how pemmican was the ultimate form of condensed food. It is prepared by adding berries to a mixture of animal fat and dried, finely pounded, lean meat in a 1:1 ratio. In this state, it said to be the "nutritional panacea" and can be preserved for lengthy periods of time. It was easily carried and provided sustenance through harsh winters.

By 1874 the hunting had reached its zenith. That year a quarter of a million hides were marketed by one trading company in Fort Macleod. Five years later that same company marketed only 5764.

In the 1920s, storyteller Peter Erasmus related to Henry Thompson his first-person experiences of the last days of the buffalo. Thompson wrote them down, and they make a compelling account of the early part of Erasmus' life during the traumatic times when the bison rapidly disappeared from the landscape of Western Canada.

Erasmus' Methodist church education led to his extraordinary career. He spoke six First Nations languages as well as English, Latin and Greek. This skill made him essential as translator of many meetings between Native peoples and British soldiers and administrators and provided him with income. His remarkable grasp of Native languages may also come from the fact that two of his forbearers, a great grandmother and a grandfather were Muscaigoe Cree.

There are many books that cover this story, including Wes Olson's, but Erasmus' account tells of the progression from successful horse-mounted hunts (in which Erasmus participated) through increasingly difficult searches to the virtual disappearance of the once main food resource of Plains People. His last buffalo hunt was in the summer of 1876. He died in 1931 at the age of 97, long since settled in a house with his family.

Both books are intriguing but ultimately sad reads about a time of huge transition.

CHAPTER 28

A Zoo Society: Yesterday and Today

I n 1976 a small group of 10 like-minded folks came up with a plan to form a zoological society in Saskatoon. Our modest goal was to support the Forestry Farm Zoo and organize monthly meetings for talks by those who would be able to entertain and inform on a wide variety of topics related to wildlife and zoos.

We advertised in the local press and got together at the vet college for our first meeting. Most of those who joined came from colleges across the university campus. Others, including Lesley Avant, joined because they were deeply interested. Claire Bullaro came on board five years later. She and Lesley have been actively involved with the society ever since.

Dr. Harry Butler from the medical school anatomy department was our first president. His field research and passion was with the lemurs of Madagascar, so his first talk drew quite a crowd. We called ourselves the Saskatoon

Regional Zoological Society. While the name was obviously intended to be all-inclusive and draw folks from the satellite towns and villages nearby, it was too pretentious and too much of a mouthful. It has been changed to The Saskatoon Zoo Society. From those 10 founding members, the membership now tops 1600.

We gradually began to take on a more active role in the politics and fundraising for the zoo. The first major new building came about after I was invited to address the local Kinsmen Club. The stories that appealed to them most were about my wildlife work in Africa. After much discussion and budget planning, they donated a large sum of money and construction began. Half a dozen enclosures on the ground floor were dedicated to small hoofed animals and eventually a wallaby arrived. The upstairs space houses glass tanks that hold fish or amphibians.

Then we approached the Kiwanis Club of Saskatoon. They are well known to be supporters of community endeavours and were soon involved in the funding, design and construction of an outdoor amphitheatre. It has served well over the years as a venue for live shows, educational programs and sheer enjoyment. Right next door, between the Kinsmen building and the amphitheatre stands a corral where friendly creatures such as pygmy goats and a dwarf Sicilian donkey are kept during summer for the children to visit and enjoy.

Turkeys and peacocks still roam the grounds of the Saskatoon zoo 40 years after my arrival, but most of the rest has changed, some for the better. Many of the paths curve more naturally, and the trees have matured and provide not only shade, but they also improve the look. The carnivore pens are built with imagination, and the atmosphere has changed enormously.

Attendance has grown steadily as improvements take place. The arrival of two white tigers, and the birth of a cub, created a huge stir and local media interest, so much so that national television and major newspapers picked up the story. Nearly 133,000 visitors flocked to the zoo that summer. That single birth caused a peak of visitor numbers that has slowly increased ever since. There is a smart new enclosure housing cougars, and a large pen with a pool holds two hand-raised grizzly bears.

Some of the livestock pens have lost their geometric shape but not all. Several of the small wooden shelters in them have hardly changed since the mid-'70s. The only innovation with these sheds is that some have small solar panels that allow a dim light inside the buildings when it is needed.

The Saskatoon Zoo Society, founded by that small group in 1976 is still active. The society has 17 employees, with numbers rising to 30 in summer when train drivers and others are in action. Lesley Avant has been an employee for 27 years. She manages the Paws Inn gift shop at the new entrance, and she ran the rather minimal concession for many years since the city chose not to improve it.

The society is really the face of the zoo, dealing with all sorts of public concerns and queries and running extensive education programs and outreach activities. A typical one is the school visits during term time. A star of those shows was the Swainson's hawk named Ariel. She had been looked after at the vet school for a while and then moved to the zoo. After 23 years going out to schools, she was recently euthanized after suffering from arthritis for many years. Hundreds of children in dozens of classrooms were fascinated by her and had the chance to learn about wild-life during her sessions in their classrooms.

The other volunteer organization that supports the facility is The Saskatoon Zoo Foundation. Working independently of the society, the foundation has raised funds for several buildings and new displays such as the Potash Corporation Ark and the Lions Event Pavilion. Another important building for which the foundation solicited funds is the Affinity Learning Centre. It is used by the society for its education programs and other events. Of late, the two organizations have merged their goals and work together on continued outreach and fund raising.

Notes on Sources

Chapter 1: New Beginnings

How Strong Is a Chimpanzee? http://www.slate.com/articles/health_and_ science/science/2009/02/how_strong_is_a_chimpanzee.html. Accessed March 30, 2015.

Chapter 3: For the Birds!

https://en.wikipedia.org/wiki/Blackstrap_Ski_Hill, Accessed May 2014.

Chapter 5: A Near Miss

T.H. White. *The Once and Future King.* William Collins, Sons. 1958.

Chapter 6: Blowgun Development

Haigh, J. *The Trouble With Lions.* Edmonton, AB: University of Alberta Press. 2008.

Chapter 8: Helicopters at –20°

"Where Men Walk With Moose." *Mutual of Omaha's Wild Kingdom.* https://www.youtube.com/watch?v=10nuKGFCXu0

Chapter 12: The Graveyard of The Atlantic

Grey Seal Breeding sounds. http://sounds.bl.uk/Environment/British- wildlife-recordings/022M-W1CDR0001378-0500V0. Accessed December 1915.

Thomas, L., M.O. Hammill, and W.D. Bowen. "Estimated size of the Northwest Atlantic grey seal population 1977–2007." Canadian Science Advisory Secretariat. Research Document 2007/082.

Zoe N. Lucas and Lisa J. Natanson. "Two shark species involved in preda- tion on seals at Sable island, Nova Scotia, Canada." Proceedings of the Nova Scotian Institute of Science (2010). Volume 45, Part 2, pp. 64–88

Fire Engine Number Four: A Battering Encounter

A.W.F. Banfield. *The Mammals of Canada.* Toronto: University of Toronto Press. 1974.

Chapter 14: A Bear Cub and a Dog

Samuel Hearne (Ken McGoogan 2007). https://www.goodreads.com/book/ show/5228147-a-journey-to-the-northern-ocean

Samuel Radbill. https://en.wikipedia.org/wiki/ Human%E2%80%93animal_breastfeeding.

Giraffe zoo cull. (http://time.com/5793/ marius-the-giraffe-not-the-only-animal-zoos-have-culled/)

Chapter 16: From Farm to Ranch

Turner ranches. http://www.tedturner.com/turner-ranches/. Accessed September 5, 2015.

Ted Turner Enterprises. http://www.tedturner.com/turner-ranches/turner- ranches-faq/. Accessed September 5, 2015.

Turner Endangered Species website. http://eowilsonfoundation.org/tag/ turner-endangered-species-fund/. Accessed September 5, 2015.

Notes on Sources

Canadian Bison Association. http://canadianbison.ca/producer/resources/data_statistics.htm. Accessed September 5, 2015.

COSEWIC bison numbers. http://www.cosewic.gc.ca/eng/sct1/searchdetail_e.cfm?id=143. Accessed September 5, 2015.

National Bison Association statistics. http://www.bisoncentral.com/about-bison/data-and-statistics. Accessed September 5, 2015.

Yellowstone bison numbers. http://www.nps.gov/yell/learn/nature/bison.htm. Accessed September 5, 2015.

Chapter 20: Scary Night

Excerpted from Interview No. IE:323 [Aipilik Innuksuk, 1995]. *Igloolik Oral History Project*, Igloolik Research Centre, Nunavut Research Institute.

MacDonald, John. *The Arctic Sky: Inuit Astronomy, Star Lore, and Legend.* Co-published by the Royal Ontario Museum and the Nunavut Research Institute. 1998.

Fire Engine Number Seven: An Outbreak and a Remedy

ABC News. *Queensland experiences doubling in salmonella cases with 1,895 reports this year so far.* http://www.abc.net.au/news/2015-03-13/salmonella-cases-more-than-double-in-queensland-in-2015/6314046. Accessed March 2015.

Salmonella Cases at AAZV conference. *Zoo Vet News.* Vol 13, 1. 1997.

Chapter 22: Déjà Vu on an Unusual Lion Case

Haigh, J.C., R.H. Keffen, D.B. Gilboe, M. Klepacki, and S.A. Chaney. "Coping Saw Blades and Pipe Cleaners as Endodontic Tools." *Journal of Zoo Animal Medicine* 13: 174. 1983.

Saskatoon Zoo Society http://www.saskatoonzoosociety.ca/. Accessed March 15, 2015.

Chapter 23: Bear Capital of the World

Ian Stirling. *Polar Bears: The Natural History of a Threatened Species.* Markham, ON: Fitzhenry & Whiteside. 2011.

Chapter 24: Rubber Bullet: A Traumatic Event

Stirling, I. *Polar Bears.* Ann Arbor, MI: University of Michigan Press. 1988.

Chapter 25: Bison Studies in Winter

Olson, W. Photographs by Johane Janelle. *Portraits of the Bison: An Illustrated Guide to Bison Society.* Edmonton, AB: University of Alberta Press. 2005.

Northwest Territories Environment and Natural Resources. "Wood Bison Management Strategy for the Northwest Territories 2010–2020."

Alberta Government: *Managing Disease Risk in Northern Alberta Wood Bison: Outside of Wood Buffalo National Park.* ISBN: 978-1-4601-4. September 2013.

Notes on Sources

Wilson G.A., C. Strobeck. "Genetic variation within and relatedness among wood and plains bison populations." Genome 42: 483–496. 1999b.

C. G. Van Zyll De Jong, C. Gates, H. Reynolds, and W. Olson. "Phenotypic Variation In Remnant Populations Of North American Bison." *Journal of Mammalogy*, Vol. 76, No. 2 (May, 1995), pp. 391–405. Published.

Fire Engine Number Nine: Preventing a Rabies Outbreak

http://www.bbc.com/news/health-33378517. Accessed July 5, 2015.

Chapter 27: Bison in Art.

Chauvet Cave Images. https://www.google.ca/search?q=Chauvet+cave+images&tbm=isch&tbo=u&source=univ&sa=X&ved=0ahUKEwi7w-JPk7MzJAhWrpIMKHXFJDVIQsAQIGw&biw=1146&bih=675. Accessed August 2012.

Clottes, J. and D. Lewis-Williams. *The Shamans of Prehistory: Trance and Magic in the Painted Caves*. New York: Harry Adamas. 1998.

Erasmus, P. *Buffalo Days and Nights*. Translated by Thompson H. Calgary, AB: Glenbow Institute. 1999.

Jerry Haigh. *Wrestling With Rhinos: The Adventures of a Glasgow Vet in Kenya*. Toronto: ECW Press. 2002.

Hammer J. *Finally, the Beauty of France's Chauvet Cave Makes its Grand Public Debut.*

http://www.smithsonianmag.com/history/france-chauvet-cave-makes-grand-debut-180954582/?no-ist Accessed April 2015.

Hertzog, W. *Cave of Forgotten Dreams.*

http://www.imdb.com/title/tt1664894/. Accessed August 2012.

Johnston, Charlie. http://www.themuralsofwinnipeg.com/MpagesSingle MuralPage.php?action=gotomural&muralid=234. Accessed July 2015.

MacEwan, G. *Buffalo Sacred and Sacrificed*. Red Deer, AB: Red Deer Press. Jan 2003.

Manitoba Museum. http://www.manitobamuseum.ca

Wes Olson. Photographs by Johane Janelle. *Portraits of the Bison: An Illustrated Guide to Bison Society*. Edmonton, AB: University of Alberta Press: 2005.

Chapter 28: A Zoo Society: Yesterday and Today

Saskatoon Zoo Society. http://saskatoonzoosociety.ca/. Accessed March 15, 2015.

Saskatoon Zoo Foundation. http://www.saskatoonzoofoundation.ca/. Accessed December 2015.

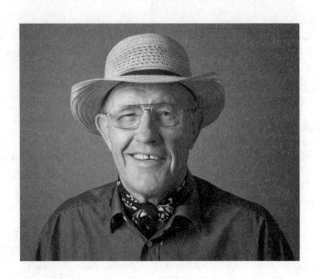

Jerry Haigh

~

Dr. Jerry Haigh is a Kenya-born, Glasgow-schooled wildlife veterinarian. He returned to Kenya three days after graduation and spent ten years there. He wrote about those experiences in his books *Wrestling With Rhinos* and *The Trouble With Lions*.

In 1975 he moved to Saskatchewan, Canada, where he continued to work with captive animals in zoos and free-ranging wildlife across the country. That work included studies of moose, caribou, seals, bison and polar bears.

He retired from the University of Saskatchewan in 2009 but continues his love of storytelling. He has told his stories across Canada from Yukon to Newfoundland, as well as in the United States and on four other continents.

To see his books, blog, wildlife photographs and wood-work projects visit him at: www.jerryhaigh.com.